Schroder Publishing

Published by Schroder Publishing.

Publisher: Daniel W. Schroder
Contact:danny@andhowtogetit.com
Copyright 2014 Daniel Wade Schroder

About the *...And How to Get It!* Series

The promise of the *...And How to Get It!* series is to empower readers with the information they need to fulfill their goals. Whether those goals involve a healthy body, a great sex life, or a self-sustaining vegetable garden, each book takes the reader on a step by step journey towards getting what they want.

Unlike comparable series of the past our books are shorter, more succinct, and better designed for today's modern book buyers. We want our readers to be able to attain what they want without all the extraneous material and filler often found in other guides. We provide the essential scoop without the fluff with concrete advice and a specific game plan. Our expert-authors are carefully selected to coach the reader through to his or her goal with the encouraging voice of experience and a wealth of knowledge behind them.

Still, the *...And How to Get It!* books are far from dull and academic. Entertainingly light and conversational with a good amount of appropriate humor, we like to sprinkle in fun bits of facts and trivia - nobody said goal attainment had to be *all* hard work! Our approach, however, is never at the expense of detouring from the topic at hand or bogging down the reader in an encyclopedic swamp of endless unusable information. We understand that the readers of today want their information provided quickly, clearly, and practically. They already know what they want or they wouldn't have selected our book in the first place. This tells us they are more than ready and anxious to dive into the process and as the author, it's your job to grab the reader's hand and help them take that first plunge beginning with page one.

Sidebars

We have included two sidebars for quick information:

GET THIS!

This sidebar presents a surprising fact the reader will find interesting within the context of what is being discussed and that will also serve to educate in an offbeat way.

GET AN EDGE!

This sidebar presents something the reader can do right now towards their goal without waiting.

We wish you the best as you discover **How to Get It!**
Daniel W. Schroder
Publisher, Schroder Publishing
www.andhowtogetit.com
danny@andhowtogetit.com

A Healthy Body

...And How to Get It!

By
Shannon Clark

ISBN: 147936102X
ISBN 13: 9781479361021

Part 1

CHAPTER 1:
The Problem With The Fitness/ Weight Loss Industry Today

Welcome to taking the very first step in achieving optimal success with your health and fitness journey. By picking up a copy of this book, you are taking action to create a better tomorrow for yourself and are getting ready to put the necessary steps in place to improve your strength, enhance your health, shed excess body weight, and learn everything that you need to know about using a proper diet and workout program.

Basically, you are creating a brand new life for yourself.

Throughout this book, we are going to cover everything that you need to know to completely transform your body so that you can see a maximum level of success.

If you've ever felt overwhelmed before when on a workout or diet plan and like you just couldn't figure out what you were doing wrong and why you weren't seeing results, that is all about to change.

After you go through this book, it's going to be very crystal clear for you and you will have the confidence you need that this will be the last plan you ever use.

My hopes are in that after using this plan, you will commit to it for life so that way you will keep up all the positive habits you are building into the future.

One of the biggest problems that is present in today's fitness industry is the strong desire for the 'quick-fix'. It seems that everyone is simply looking to get results – yesterday – and they are willing to do whatever it takes to achieve those results, even if it means forgoing proper health in the process.

This is a big problem.

Remember, nothing is more important than your health here.

After all, this is why we are putting forth the plan that we are – to improve your health. Improved appearance and body composition are just going to be a byproduct of the enhanced health results you will receive.

But this means that you must be focusing on a permanent change here, not a quick fix that has you doing everything under the sun to drop body weight, which often isn't even body fat, but rather water weight or even worse, muscle mass tissue.

This is not what you want.

Focus on the right approach and believe me, you will fare far better. The biggest problem today is that people are simply not willing to give the effort they should be to construct a proper diet and workout program.

But, by reading this book, you're showing that you are already one step ahead of the rest of those people and are going against the norm.

You want to acquire the information that will help you proceed forward. You don't just want to read a plan and start up imme-diately. You want to learn the why's of what you're doing.

And trust me, those why's – they will help bring you success.

When you're struggling and fee like tossing in the towel, knowing the why's is what will help you carry onward and choose otherwise.

So what are we going to cover in this book?

First we're going to take a look at the top mistakes that people make as they go about their diet protocol. If you can learn what not to do, this will help you make sure that you are doing the right things to see success.

After that, we're going to talk about what it means for you to be healthy. Different people have different definitions, so this is important to get straight as well.

From there, we'll cover how to master your mindset so that you are setting yourself up for success. How you think as you go about this program – and the things you are saying to yourself, will make a big difference in whether you stick with it, so this cannot be overlooked.

We'll also talk about goal setting and what you must do there to ensure your success.

From that section, we'll move on to the theory section and talk about why both exercise and diet are vital for success.

Then we'll cover the in's and out's of building a proper diet including setting your target calorie intake, making sure your macronutrients are lined up for success, and designing a plan that you can actually stick with for life. Remember, adherence is our number one priority, so we are going to do everything possible to ensure you stay the course over time.

We'll also go over how to make smart choices when you eat out so that you are sure to maintain a proper diet plan. If you don't choose wisely here, it can be incredibly detrimental to your progress.

From there, we'll give you some tips on getting past any plateau that you encounter so if progress ever does get slow, you know precisely what to do.

After that, we'll go over the in's and out's of exercise – the different forms of exercise you can do and the benefits of each along with the factors that come into play when designing a workout program.

We'll also go over what you need to get into place if you want to design a proper home gym. It's important to consider where you will feel best doing your workout as this can influence your adherence as well.

Then we'll finish up by talking about overtraining and what you need to know about that. If you want to stay committed and on track, you must avoid overtraining at all costs.

After that, we'll move into the last part of the book where we will give you your diet and workout plans so that you can get started immediately.

At that point you will have everything that you need to move forward and start seeing the results that you're looking for.

So if you're ready, let's get our discussion kick-started and go over the biggest mistakes that many people make with their diet and workout program.

CHAPTER 2:
The Top Mistakes People Make When Trying To Get Fit And Healthy

So you've just set the goal to lose weight and firm up. You're feeling great! You've taken the steps to find a program that you think will work and are ready to give 110% of your full effort.

You are anticipating great results this time around because you feel confdient that this is the program that is going to deliver.

But is it really?

In far too many cases, it isn't.

Even the smallest of mistakes in some cases can completely send you off track with you results and for some people, off the fitness and health enhancement bandwagon entirely.

So we're going to walk you through the top ten of these mistakes right now so that you can feel certain you are not committing these fatal sins.

Mistake #1: Overdoing Cardio Training

When many people set out on the goal to lose fat, the very first thing they do is run straight to the cardio machines. They figure, the more cardio training they can get in, the faster they are going to be moving to their end goal.

So they run on that treadmill or cycle away on that bike like a hamster on a wheel. Morning and night – they are in the gym as often as they can be 'doing their time' on the cardio machines.

And while don't get me wrong, some cardio training can and most likely should be part of a well-balanced fitness program, this is entirely the wrong way to go about things.

If you find yourself doing more than an hour or two *total* of cardio training per week, you can now classify yourself as a 'cardio bunny' – as these people are often called.

There are numerous problems with doing this much cardio training.

First, you're going to find that boredom sets in quickly. Let's face the facts, doing hours on end of cardio training is not fun, or enjoyable. Sure, it may be if you decide to tune into your nightly TV shows or catch up on the latest gossip in the celebrity magazine that's now a mandatory requirement of any cardio session, but if this is the case, let's be real here – how hard are you actually working?

If you can read a magazine while you're doing cardio training, you aren't working all that hard.

Second, and possibly the bigger problem with all this cardio training is that it's not particular challenging for the body.

If you want to change the way your body looks and get fitter, you need to give your body a reason to need to change.

Doing a form of exercise that you can easily complete without any issues is not giving your body a reason at all.

In fact, it's just encouraging your body to stay the same.

Plus, with so much low resistance cardio training, you'll be more likely to lose lean muscle mass, which is the complete opposite of what you want here.

If you start losing lean muscle mass, you're going to look less toned and defined than before, your strength level is going to go down, and the absolute worst thing about this – your metabolic rate will start to get slower.

Remember, muscle is highly metabolically active tissue, meaning the more of it you have, the more calories you are going to burn each day to simply stay alive. This is a big reason why men seem to maintain their body weight more easily than women – or they can eat more food without fat gain.

They have a greater amount of lean muscle mass burning up calories daily, helping keep them lean.

So if you go doing all those hours on the treadmill and start losing muscle because of it, what do you think this will mean for your future fat loss progress?

It means the outlook is grim.

If you're moving your body across such great distances however (as you are when you're doing your cardio training), you are basically telling your body that it needs to learn to be as fuel efficient as possible.

Endurance training does take a decent amount of energy and in order to survive these sessions, the body knows that the fewer calories it burns, the better.

Since muscle burns so many calories at rest, it's the first tissue to go.

Finally, the last problem with doing all this cardio training in your program is that it means there isn't going to be much time for anything else. You'll be so caught up in doing your hours and hours of cardio training that even trying to fit in more productive forms of exercise (such as weight lifting – more on this later), won't be happening.

So the first mistake you must avoid at all costs is overdoing the cardio training element of things.

Do this and you can count on moving backwards.

Mistake #2: Crash Dieting

The second mistake that you absolutely must be avoiding is crash dieting. This happens far too often in the diet industry. Someone sees a quick-fix diet that promises that if you just use it, you can lose 10 pounds in 10 days.

Or, maybe you're going to melt 5 inches in two weeks.

Whatever the claim is, you're hungry for results and jump right to it.

Bad move.

Crash dieting is no way to reach a healthy body weight.

There are so many problems associated with crash dieting, that I'm not even sure where to start.

First, it's not healthy, but you likely don't need me to tell you that (hopefully!). Your body requires so many vitamins and minerals each and every day and if you are not providing these, problems are going to occur.

But, being able to provide these nutrients in sufficient quantities takes food – and calories.

If you're eating 600 a day, how is that going to happen?

It's not and you will be feeling miserable in no time. Sure, you may be able to take a multi-vitamin and get some back up support, but nutrients are always better coming from food and even with that multi, you may still not get everything you need.

In the short term, it may be fine, but it is no long term solution.

The next and more critical reason why these crash diets are not the way to a better body is because you have built in mechanisms that are going to fight back against a very low calorie diet that you are just not going to be able to fight.

You see, your body has its own goal in mind. it's called *survival*.

 Get an Edge!
To get a quick approximately of the bare minimum number of calories you should consume, multiply your current body weight by 10. Don't go any lower than this.

The minute you put yourself on a very low calorie diet approach, your body is realizing that there is definitely not much fuel coming in and sees this as an emergency situation. It doesn't realize that you just want to fit into your size 4 'skinny jeans' or that you simply want to have some shredded abs for the beach, it thinks there is a famine taking place and is going to do everything and anything it can to make sure that you stay alive.

There are a number of hormones involved in the process that will take place, but the end result is that you will start feeling miserable.

You'll be exhausted (moving is enough work, never mind *exercising!*)

You'll have an insatiable hunger level.

Your metabolic rate will plummet.

You'll be irritable.

You'll feel freakishly cold all the time.

Basically, your body is trying to get you to do nothing but eat and sleep. Sleep is when your calorie burn drops the lowest, so it makes sense that your body would want you to do this. You're then conserving fuel as best as possible. The fewer calories you burn, the longer you can stay alive in spite of such little food intake.

Now trust me, when you are in a war with your body, you are not going to come out ahead. These feelings are just going to be too strong to fight, even if you have iron-like will power. You will cave, and when you do, chances are you will go on a week-long binge because you've felt so deprived.

This is also precisely why you see so many of those people who use crash diets falling off them after a week or two and then gaining not only the weight they lost right back, *but then some.*

Clearly this is a very bad thing.

What's more is that because your metabolism slows down so significantly while you are taking in so few calories, this then means that when you come off that crash diet and begin shoveling food frantically into your mouth (because let's face it, this is what most people do if we're downright honest), your body is primed for *fat gain.*

Slow metabolism + high calorie diet.

I don't think I need to spell that one out for you.

So hopefully now you can see just why those crash diets need to be a thing of your past.

If you want to get leaner and healthier – and stay that way forever, a crash diet is by no means your solution.

The sooner you can accept this and learn to stay away from these altogether, the better.

Mistake #3: Going To Any Sort Of Extremes

Next up we have another related issue and that is going to extremes of any kind. If you're on a program that has you completely eliminating a certain form of nutrient – either a zero carb approach or a diet that requires all food to have 'fat-free' behind the name, you're headed for disaster.

Not only are extremist approaches like this going to leave you devoid in nutrients as each main nutrient does provide nutrients your body needs on a regular basis, but they are going to leave you feeling miserable as well.

If you're not eating any carbohydrates for example, you're going to likely find that your energy level tanks as carbohydrates are the main source of fuel for your body.

On the other hand, if you're not eating any dietary fats, you'll likely find that you're starving all throughout the day because the addition of dietary fats to your meals is what makes them 'stick to your ribs', so to speak.

If you aren't eating enough dietary fats, you'll get hungry very shortly after eating each meal, so this too is definitely going to work against you.

Not to mention that you may start to find that your diet overall tastes a little bit like cardboard due to the fact that fats add flavor and moisture.

There are many other reasons of course that these nutrients need to be added – health reasons, which we will discuss when we get to the macronutrient section, but for now just note that if you're eating a diet that has you at any extreme, you're not on a diet that is going to yield good results.

Balance is key.

Balance keeps you healthy, happy, and seeing results.

Mistake #4: Exercising As Much As Possible

The next mistake that is commonly made goes hand in hand with the last mistake and that is exercising as much as you possibly can.

If you think that the more exercise you do, the faster you will lose fat, you've got another thing coming. This is a very incorrect notion that far too many people believe and they just land themselves in trouble because of it.

We've already discussed the fact that too much cardio is very detrimental to your results, but too much exercise – whatever variety you happen to be using – is also going to be bad news if you want to see optimal results.

If you do too much exercise on your approach, your body views this in a very similar nature to using too low of a calorie intake.

Either way, you're expending far more calories than what you're consuming on a day to day basis and this is definitely going to be cause for concern.

And if you decide to really go at things and use a very low calorie intake coupled with a very high volume workout program, now you're definitely asking for trouble.

The body must have enough rest each week for results to occur.

What you must remember here is that it's during the rest period where you're actually making progress.

When you're in the gym, you're actually just breaking your body down, so results will not be seen.

When you're outside the gym, that's when you're building your body back up, growing stronger than you were before.

So if you hit the gym too often, you'll actually just keep tearing down those muscle tissues before they've had a chance to grow back stronger and you can imagine what this means for your progress moving forward.

You'll start getting weaker and losing muscle mass tissue.

Basically, the opposite of what you want to have happen will happen.

In addition to this, too much exercise will also just burn you out. You'll be feeling exhausted all the time and your motivation to get those workout sessions in will be so low that they likely won't happen for much longer.

Exercise, like your diet, needs to be balanced.

Rest is a vital component of any well-designed workout program.

 Get an Edge!
If your health care plan provides for it, get one deep tissue massage per week. This can go a long way towards speeding up the entire recovery process.

Mistake #5: Relying Too Heavily On Supplements

Next, we've all met those people – the ones who are constantly chasing the next best supplement to get them to their end goal.

They read about such and such product online or in some magazine and next thing you know, they're buying themselves a few bottles.

When that one doesn't produce results, they're onto the newest thing that's come out since.

On and on the cycle continues.

What you must realize here is that supplements are just that. They are designed to *supplement* your program, not replace it.

They don't call them replacements for a reason. If you are relying too heavily on supplementation and thinking that if you take the right supplement you won't need to put in the work necessary to make good progress, you're going to be in for disappointment.

Not to mention that the sad fact is that many of the supplements that people will gravitate to – those that do promise quick-fix results, are the ones that could put your health at risk if you aren't careful because they aren't natural in any manner.

When looking at supplements to use on your program, you want to do your best to choose supplements that are nutrients in themselves. So in this case, you'd want to choose something like fish oil if you aren't meeting your omega fat intake.

Or, you might choose to supplement with vitamin D if you aren't getting enough sun or vitamin D enriched foods.

Supplements that promise to boost your metabolism, burn fat for you, block the absorption of fat or carbs (never a good thing!) or otherwise are not the ones that you want to be leaning towards.

Yes, there are definitely supplements out there that can enhance your energy level to a relatively good degree and there are also supplements out there that may assist with appetite control as well, but they aren't going to perform miracles.

You simply cannot expect a supplement to do the work for you.

You must put in the time and effort with your overall diet and workout protocol to see results and the sooner you can accept this, the sooner success will be yours.

Mistake #6: Expecting Instant Results

The next mistake that's often made is the simple mistake of lack of patience. You put yourself on a program and expect to be seeing physical changes in one week's time.

One week is enough you figure – you should be seeing results.

Realize that while some people may start to see some results occurring after the first week, this is more the exception than the rule.

It takes time for significant changes to occur and if you're expecting immediate progress, the chances that you are going to be thrown off course as your motivation plummets when you aren't is going to be pretty high.

While you may see a significant drop in the scale during the first week on a diet plan, you must realize that most often this is simply water weight you're losing and not true body weight.

After that initial week is up and the rush of weight loss is gone, your results will slow down.

The good news though is that if you're following a well-designed program, such as this one, then you will be losing *fat* at this point, not water.

While water weight is great and can give you a nice little boost to your motivation since you're now looking leaner, it would come back on just as quickly if you came off that diet plan.

By adopting the right frame of mind, which we will talk into great detail on in the coming chapter, you can make sure that you are not going to be easily swayed off course if you don't see results in a few days.

Lack of commitment, perseverance, and motivation is the number one reason why far too many people do not get the results that they are hoping for.

Good things come to those who wait – remember this and live by it.

This isn't to say that it'll take years for you to see progress (at least not if you use this program), but you must get over your need for instant gratification.

If you work hard, persist, and bounce back despite any setbacks that do occur, you will be heavily rewarded.

Mistake #7: Neglecting Strength Training

Now we come to another fatal workout sin, which is neglecting strength training altogether.

This one does tend to be a bit more common in women than men as they fear getting 'bulky'.

Let's lay that fear to rest.

What all the women who are reading this right now need to realize is that the chances of you getting 'bulky' or looking too manly is about 0.0000000000001%.

I'm completely serious.

Women do not possess the level of testosterone in their body to build up significant amounts of lean muscle mass, so if you think that getting bulky is in your cards, you better think again.

You will build muscle at a fraction of the rate a man would and generally speaking, it is very hard for women to accumulate a decent amount of muscle mass.

In fact, most women would be lucky to gain around 5-6 pounds of muscle *per year.*

Add to this that building muscle takes eating more calories and many women out there are on a perpetually low calorie intake, so that also adds a big boulder to the 'get bulky' equation.

It just won't happen.

Plus, you must remember that you are in control here. Even if you do start to feel like you're at the point where you don't want any more muscle, you can stop building more muscle right then and there.

It's completely up to you.

You will not, trust me, wake up one morning and look like a man.

Instead, strength training is going to help you look leaner, tighter, fitter, and if you perform strength training correctly, it'll enhance all the feminine curves you have on your body as well.

Furthermore, as we'll get into a little bit later, strength training is by far the best exercise for boosting your metabolic rate, meaning by doing it, you can become a fat fighting machine.

Those who strength train will be far less likely to deal with weight gain as time progresses onwards, so that's yet another reason why they shouldn't fear this variety of workout.

Strength training is a must.

Most men will gravitate to strength training more than anything else, so we don't need to have the same discussion for them, however if you are one of those few males who chooses not to do it for whatever reason, it's time for you to start.

Get This!

Those who strength train are more likely to lose weight and keep it off for good than those who do cardio training. So if you had to choose between both of these, strength training should be your choice!

Mistake #8: Never Allowing Indulgence

The next mistake that's often made as people go about their programs to lose weight and firm up is never allowing for any indulgence at all.

While it's definitely going to be very important that you are scratching a number of foods off your regular eating list, there's no reason to completely avoid all foods that you enjoy.

If you can remember to make it about a 90/10% split between eating healthy and on-program and 10% having a bit more fun and enjoying what you crave, you're going to sustain a much more positive relationship with food that will ensure that you don't start to get a little too obsessive.

We've all likely experienced this problem before.

As soon as you say that you cannot eat X and X food, those are the foods that you start thinking about non-stop.

You obsess about them – some people might even dream about them.

When you simply put a food on the 'for later' list, this problem doesn't occur. Now you know you can have it and your cravings will be satisfied, you'll just have to wait a little while for that to happen.

This is a big difference in the mindset of a dieter and an important one.

Furthermore, another big problem with those who put foods on the 'never eat' list is the fact that you'll be using black and white thinking patterns.

So basically, if you do give in to temptation and eat one of those foods on your never list, you feel like you've completely failed entirely and are far more likely to give up entirely and go on a full out food binge.

What started out as one or two cookies to satisfy your craving turns into a box of cookies – and in some cases, a tub of ice cream to boot.

If this happens, now you're talking trouble. While a few cookies may have set you back slightly in progress, a box of cookies plus a tub of ice cream will do you in.

You'll have easily undone a week's worth of hard work for 10 minutes of some good-food-eating.

Those who don't use black and white thinking, who don't have this good/bad, yes/no set-up going on are far more likely to be able to get past that smaller indulgence of just a cookie or two.

They'll realize that it wasn't the best choice, but will be able to chalk it up to a mistake and move forward.

Get This!
Those who never cheat on their diet are less likely to see success because they will develop a very bad relationship with food and may actually develop an eating disorder over time. Learn that all foods have a healthy place in your diet.

In that scenario, it'll just be a small bump in the road to greater success.

So it really pays to start giving more attention to your frame of mind surrounding food.

By having planned 'cheat' days in your program, you'll learn how to incorporate the foods that you may not normally eat without losing complete control and come to see that you won't gain back 10 pounds overnight if you do choose to eat them.

They can easily be incorporated into a sound diet plan and keep you moving along towards your end goal.

Mistake #9: Not Tracking Progress

Now we come to the next mistake and that mistake is failing to track your progress. If you're not tracking the progress that you're making, this could come to impact you in a number of ways.

First, you won't get the motivational boost that tracking provides. If you're tracking your body weight/fat level, your amount of weight lifted, the time you take between sets, and so on, you're going to be seeing clear progress being made and this is very inspiring to help you to keep pushing onward.

Those who track everything will have a clear record to look back on and at times, that simple refresher is precisely what you need to give yourself a jump-start to keep going.

The second reason that tracking is so important is because this will also allow you to better pinpoint why you may or may not be seeing success.

If you aren't getting results with your fat loss diet for instance, then you know that chances are good you may be taking in too many calories.

To help improve the situation so that you start losing weight again, you would decrease your calorie intake slightly so that you were taking in fewer.

If you weren't tracking, how would you know what to consume? There'd be no record of how many calories you were eating so you'd have no way to judge this.

Finally, tracking helps you make sure that you are making progress with your workouts.

While some people may just have a very good memory and might be able to remember the exact weight they lifted along with how many reps were performed and how must rest was taken, most won't.

Next time you go into the gym, it is important that you do a little more than you did last time and a clear record of what was done ensures that you do actually do so.

Tracking may take a little bit more time out of your day to get done, but that time will be very well spent.

Mistake #10: Not Setting Proper Goals

Finally, the last mistake that many people make on their quest for a healthier and fit body is not setting proper goals in the first place.

We'll be talking much more about goal setting in a coming chapter, but for now you need to realize that setting proper goals will be paramount if you are going to sustain good motivation and see the results you're after.

This involves both how your goals are formulated as well as the number and types of goals that you set.

If either of these is off in any way, you're starting off on the wrong foot.

By taking the time to ensure that you do set proper goals however, you can feel confident that you will be moving in the right direction from the start.

Most people when setting their goals just think of the main thing that they want to accomplish and that's that.

These goals are not defined at all, they're not specific enough, and often times, they are going to be too far off in the distance to really keep you feeling inspired and motivated to carry on.

We'll cover proper goal setting shortly, so you won't need to worry about that.

So there you have the main problems that you may find yourself facing and that will lead you to significant trouble in terms of moving forward and seeing the results that you're looking for.

If you can make sure that you are doing everything possible to avoid these mistakes, you can feel good that you aren't committing a fatal sin that will cost you your time, energy, and end goals.

So now that this is out of the way, let's move onward and talk about how to master your mindset so that you are moving in the right direction from the start.

CHAPTER 3:
Defining Your Own Version Of What Healthy Means

When you hear the term 'healthy', what comes to mind? What do you think it takes for you to personally consider yourself healthy?

Everyone has a different version of what healthy means to them and it's important that you take the time to learn what that means to you so that you know precisely what you are after with this program plan.

After all, if you don't have a clear vision in place, how will you know what you're after? How will you have the direction you need?

It's simple – you won't.

So take some time right now and think about what your definition of healthy is.

Is it having more energy?

Feeling stronger and being able to accomplish everyday activities and tasks that much easier?

Is it knowing that you are at a lower disease risk because of the steps you are taking to ensure a healthy body?

Or perhaps being healthy is about creating a stress free lifestyle that gives you peace of mind. Maybe you feel that when you are looking after your body you can relax in knowing that you are going to be strong and viable for years to come.

For other people, being healthy isn't just about fitness or your body weight, but about a lifestyle choice that means doing the things you enjoy and maintaining an active social life.

Remember, being 'healthy' doesn't always involve body health, but can also encompass mental health as well.

If your mind isn't healthy, that's a big problem as well as the mind and body go together.

Likewise, your soul needs to be healthy as well. If you don't feel fulfilled in your day to day life, this can also be a big problem and prevent you from accomplishing what you want as you move through the years. You won't have the desire and determination you might otherwise would and may find that you lack the commitment for personal growth.

Being healthy is different for everyone but if you stop and think about what your own personal definition of healthy is, you can then tailor your program to match.

If you're someone who values social well-being as much as fitness, you may schedule fewer workouts over the course of the week so you have more time to spend with friends doing social activities you enjoy.

Likewise, if you're someone who values being mentally healthy, perhaps you enroll in some evening classes to learn a new skill along with doing a few workouts a week.

While this book is primarily going to cover the fitness and nutrition aspects of being healthy, note that as you make the changes in these two areas, you must not neglect other areas of your life that you feel are also required for you to be healthy.

Take the most comprehensive approach as you possibly can and that will ensure that you end up seeing the long-term results and success that you're after.

To help you take this one step forward and get your mind in the right place, let's now move and talk more about how you can prepare for success by getting your mindset set up as you should.

CHAPTER 4:
Mindset Mastery – Preparing For Success

Getting into the right frame of mind is going to be one of the most important elements that you must do if you want to move forward and see the success that you're after.

Far too many people are impacted by negative goals, negative thought patterns, and negative self-statements that the chances of them actually seeing progress is about zero to none.

If you take a few steps before you start however to get your frame of mind set up for success, this doesn't have to impact you in this manner.

Let's first begin our discussion with proper goal setting and then we'll move onto talk about self-statements, the importance of visualization, as well as other motivational techniques that you'll want to consider.

 Get an Edge!
Take some time to get yourself a goals journal. Find one that's small enough that you can carry it around regularly so that you can constantly update your goals at any time of the day.

How To Set Proper Goals

The very first thing that you need to make sure that you're taking into account is proper goal setting. If you aren't setting good goals before you begin, you won't have a clear path of where you're going.

It would be similar to trying to travel somewhere without having a road map or directions. You'd likely get lost along the way and rather than reaching your end goal, you'd end up traveling around and around in circles, becoming more frustrated with each and every lap that you made.

The thing to know about goal setting is that it's never finished. While you will set your goals before you get started and that will be that, you need to be constantly re-evaluating these goals and making sure that they are still applicable where you're at and are going to serve you well moving into the future.

If you aren't doing this re-evaluation, you might find yourself following goals that just don't apply any longer and then you'll really be moving a step in the wrong direction.

Goals should be reviewed and read through each week. This will not only keep you hungrier since you will know what it is that you are working towards, but it'll help ensure that you are working toward what you want to be working toward.

Why waste time on a goal that's no longer important? Life changes and in some cases, what was important for you to be achieving before will no longer be something that you're concerned with in the future.

Now, when formulating your goals, it's a good idea to use the SMART goal setting concept.

Let's look at what this entails.

Specific

First, the goal needs to be specific. As we just mentioned, don't state that you want to 'lose weight'. That's not good enough.

How much do you want to lose?

Better yet, how much body fat do you want to shed? Remember, losing weight and losing body fat can mean different things. Your mission is to lose body fat – not lean muscle mass.

By focusing on this, you'll do far better.

On the flip side, it may be muscle building you're after. If this is the case, how much muscle do you want to build? Get a definite amount in place so that you have a clear path of focus.

Measurable

Second, you also need to make sure whatever goal you set is measurable as well. If you've set a goal that's very specific, it should be, by nature, measurable as well.

There are some weight loss and health oriented goals that may not be all that measurable – improving your confidence for example. It's hard to know exactly when this is reached as it's more of a process than anything.

If you've set some immeasurable goals, just be sure that you do have a few that are measurable as well.

Think decreases in body fat, decreases in measurements, fitting into a certain size, or improvements in specific health readings that you can measure (your blood pressure, for example).

Attainable

Next up, you also must make sure the goal you have set is attainable. Is this something that you could possibly do?

Don't set your sights on a goal that's simply out of reach. For example, if you're currently 180 pounds, 5'10" and have never been lower than 140, don't set the goal to get down to 120. Chances are that's just a little too lofty for you.

You can't fight the natural make-up of your body so you need to learn what is attainable and what's simply not.

Contrary to what you may believe, we are not all cut out to look like supermodels.

Realistic

In addition to making sure your goal is attainable, also make sure it's realistic.

Many people often get realistic confused with attainable. Attainable refers to whether or not you can actually ever attain that goal. Is it possible for you? That's the basic question you're answering.

With realistic, you're asking the question of whether that goal is something you could achieve given the resources and time frame you have available to you.

For example, losing 20 pounds may be very attainable for you. Losing 20 pounds in one week…that's likely not so realistic.

So you must make sure your goal is both attainable as well as realistic. Make sure you are very honest with yourself in this section as far too many people will begin to overestimate just how much time they have to spend on their workouts or what they are willing to do diet-wise.

But then when push comes to shove, they realize that they aren't quite willing to do what they had thought they would, and as such, their goal is no longer realistic.

Think about the efforts you've given in the past and bump them up just a small amount – don't go expecting a miracle from yourself because chances are, it's not going to happen.

Timeline

Finally, the last element that must be in place with your goals is that it has a firm timeline. This basically refers to when you want to accomplish the goal by.

Don't set your timeline too short that you'll be stressed out if you miss a beat, but don't set it too far off in the future that you can easily procrastinate for quite some time without worry.

Remember that life will always happen and there will be days where things just don't go as planned. A workout or two may be skipping and this is perfectly normal and natural.

As long as you do have a bit of leeway built into your plan however to account for these times, this shouldn't cause an incredible upset to your results.

A smart timeline will keep you attending the gym and sticking with your diet. It's also helpful to tell someone about your timeline so that you do feel you will be held accountable to this deadline.

Have them check in with you ever so often and see how you're doing. This way, you'll feel more compelled to actually do it because you'll have to answer to someone.

If there's no one holding you accountable, why should you care?

Who's going to stop you from not going forward and doing the program?

For many people, their own accountability is just not enough, as sad as that may be. They need an external source of accountability in place to get results.

So there you have the five things that a good goal must possess for it to help you out with your journey.

If the goals you've set don't follow in line with these, it may be time to reconsider them.

Another thing that you want to try and get into place is both process goals as well as outcome goals.

What's the difference?

Basically, a process goal is a goal that is going to be reached through *doing*.

An outcome goal is the goal that is reached *because* of all that doing.

So for example, eating five servings of vegetables per day would be a process goal because it involves you doing something specific.

Losing five pounds, in part because you choose to eat those vegetables rather than chocolate, is the outcome goal.

It's what your process goals led to.

By having process goals in place, you'll be able to break down that outcome goal so that it feels more attainable.

Process goals give you something to focus on in the here and now – they're more short term oriented and something that you can do today, not something that you will reach weeks or months down the road.

Think of them as mini-goals if you will, stepping stones along your path.

One very good technique to use with your goal setting is to set one or two process goals each day when you wake up.

 Get an Edge!

If it helps you, set two small goals for each day of the week on Sunday. This way, you don't have to think about it – you can just look at your goal journal and you're ready to start.

As your alarm sounds and you lay there, rather than wishing you could just have 10 more minutes of sleeping and thinking about your mountain to-do list for the day (which is only going to want to make you stay in bed longer!), take some time to think about three things that you want to do that very day.

Three things that you will feel good about doing when you lie back down in your bed to go to sleep, knowing that they have helped move you in the right direction.

I cannot even begin to tell you how empowering this process will be, especially for those of you who have really struggled in the past to reach goals you've set.

If that describes you, chances are very high that you have severely damaged self-beliefs. We'll talk more about self-beliefs in a second, but basically, you don't believe in yourself fully and completely.

While you may *hope* you can do it, you're still not quite sure.

You've failed so many times in the past, that you're a little timid that you'll actually be able to see results here.

But, by setting each of these three small process goals *and accomplishing them,* when you do lie in bed that evening, you will feel incredibly.

You'll feel strong.

You'll feel powerful.

You'll feel like you <u>can and will</u> accomplish what you desire.

And the even better news, the more often you do this, the stronger these feelings will get.

Pretty soon, your confidence in your ability to achieve your long term goals will be soaring and there will be no doubt in your mind that you will get results.

The mind is an incredibly powerful thing and you may have heard before that 'what you think will often come true'.

This is very often the case.

If you think that you'll never have success, the chances are mighty high that you won't.

If you think that you will, on the other hand, well then you might just surprise yourself when you're walking away reaching your end goal in due time.

Process goals will help you believe in yourself so make sure that you are setting them.

Give each day a purpose when you wake up that morning.

Now that goal setting is covered, let's move on and talk a little more about the importance of self-talk.

Looking Closely At Your Self-Talk

Next you need to start looking at the self-talk that you're using. This includes all the things that you're saying to yourself on a day to day basis that could be influencing your own self-beliefs in your ability to see success.

Most people are constantly talking to themselves on a daily basis, but few ever take the time to tune into what they are saying – or give it the credit that it deserves.

If you're saying negative self-statements to yourself, constantly berating your own capabilities to reach the goals that you've set for yourself, how do you think this will influence your desire to move forward?

If when you should be doing things one way you are instead warning yourself not to do something entirely else, will you be able to come through and do what you're supposed to?

Rather than focusing on what you shouldn't be doing, you should be focusing on what you should be doing, but when you're using a high amount of negative self-talk, focusing on what you should be doing isn't happening.

Negative self-talk will come back to damage yourself self-esteem, your self- perseverance to move forward, as well as your self-efficacy (belief in your capabilities).

You'll be in a negative frame of mind and once you're there, that is very hard to overcome.

Being in a negative frame of mind is going to do absolutely nothing to helping keep you motivated.

For example, think back to when you were in high school or university. If you continually kept telling yourself that you would never get good marks and that it was impossible to get an A in a particular class, why would you even feel compelled to try?

You'd feel defeated before you even got started.

The same principles apply here. If you aren't saying positive self-statements that encourage you to try harder and help strengthen your belief that you can achieve results, you're not going to put forth the effort that you should be.

So then, lack of effort becomes your real problem here. With low amounts of effort, you definitely won't be getting results – there's no doubt about that.

To help remedy this situation, for the next few days, start paying more attention to each and every thing that you are saying to yourself.

Start really listening in so that you can hear the words being said and give them the attention they deserve.

Then, whenever you hear yourself saying a negative self-statement about yourself, flip that negative statement into two positive statements.

At first this may be hard and you might even feel a little bit funny doing it, but if you keep pushing through and doing this process, it will have a tremendous influence on your rate of success as well as your motivation.

 Get an Edge!
Start noting your self-talk and writing those statements down in a journal. When you see them on paper, it's easier to recognize just how inaccurate these beliefs really are.

Even better, once you start the process of being more aware of what you are telling yourself, you'll be that much more aware moving forward as well. You'll naturally listen to yourself and catch yourself in negative thought patterns before they get too far, flipping them around so that they are more positive and favorable.

For those of you who are really struggling with this concept, it might also help to jot down a good 10-20 positive things about yourself before you even start so that you have some statements already built-up and ready to go when you find those negative thoughts creeping in.

Self-talk is a big deal, so make sure yours is working for you, not against you.

Now let's move on and talk about one particular technique that can be very helpful for improving your drive for success.

Harnessing The Power Of Visualization

One of the most powerful motivational techniques that you can use to kick-start a sluggish motivation level is visualization.

This technique is very often also used by top level Olympic athletes, so as you can imagine, it is one that is going to produce results.

There are two main ways you can go about using visualizations. The first is to simply use it to boost your hunger and desire to go after the goals that you have set for yourself.

Second, you can also use it whenever you have a particular event coming up that you feel like you may not be able to get through while maintaining your program plan, such as a dinner party, a large get together, or anything else of that nature.

These types of events do tend to throw people off their plan far more often than not, so preparing yourself a bit beforehand is a must.

Let's look at how to use visualizations in each of these circumstances.

The first thing that you'll want to do, regardless of the reason you are using the visualizations is to find somewhere quiet to lie.

You want to be somewhere that you will be undisturbed for at least 10-15 minutes so that you can get your visualizations completed and in without distraction. They are going to require you to focus in on intense thought patterns, so if you're disrupted, it can throw the entire process off.

Once you've found this space, then you are to lay down, close your eyes and feel your body relaxing. Many people find that it helps to contract each muscle tightly and then relax it as they feel the stress and tension flow out of their body.

Do this for 2-3 minutes and then once you're feeling fully relaxed, you can begin your visualizations.

For the first variation of the visualization, you will want to picture yourself at your end goal. Imagine what it will be like when you reach that end goal.

How will you feel?

How will others react around you?

What areas – if any – of your life are different now that you're at that end goal?

The more you can really be in that moment, feeling fully what it's like, the stronger this technique is going to be for you. You'll really be able to get a taste of success and that taste, when you then come out of the visualization, is what will drive you to keep pushing forward.

Your hunger for success will be that much greater and you'll want to keep pushing the barrier to see progress.

In essence, it's like giving a child a toy to play with and then taking it away. If you do this, they are going to try with all their might to get that toy back – it's all they'll focus on.

The same thing goes here. Give yourself a quick peek at success and then when you return back to reality, your hunger will be much stronger.

If you do this on a semi-weekly or weekly basis, you will maintain the level of desire that you need.

The second way in which you can use those visualizations is to get past any hurdle that you may face.

By imaging yourself getting through that event successfully, doing exactly what you need, you will increase the chances that you actually do so in real life.

Experience makes us stronger and allows us to learn how to better achieve success. By using the visualization here, you're essentially giving yourself that experience that you need.

Even though it is just visualizations, it's still going to factor in to building up your self-esteem to getting you through that hurdle that you are going to face.

If you can do these visualizations a couple of times before you are going to be attending that event, you be feeling far surer of yourself going in.

So there you have what you need to know about the power of visualizations. If you often find yourself struggling with motivation, they are definitely one of the best techniques to start including on a regular basis as you move throughout your program plan.

Now let's go on and talk more about some of the top motivational tips to remember as you go forward.

Motivational Techniques To Stay Committed

Now that we've talked about the importance of and how to go about your visualization practices, it's also important to take a closer look at some of the other motivational techniques that you can be using to take your progress up a notch.

Once again, if you're someone who does tend to struggle with motivation and know that this is in fact the case for you, then you're best bet is to go in prepared.

If you're doing some motivational strategies from the start, you can reduce the chances that it ever has to be an issue for you.

This said, keep in mind that what motivates one person may not necessarily motivate another, so making sure that they are personalized for you is also essential for your success.

Let's look at the main ones that you should be considering.

Getting A Program Partner

The first tip to help yourself stay motivated is to get a program partner. This could be someone who is going to be doing the diet with you, or alternatively, join you for your workouts each day.

In an ideal world, but depending on their own personal goals, that may not happen. Either way, as long as you have them join you for at least one element of the program plan, you can see positive benefits because of it.

On the diet front, they'll be there for you during those hard times when you just feel like tossing in the towel and forgoing any further work. You two can air your grievances to each other and this will, without a doubt, be a great way to release the pent up stress and tension that you're feeling and feel more compelled to keep going forward.

Sometimes all you need is a good vent session and having someone to listen to you can really work in your favor.

Get an Edge!
Those who have social support are much more likely to not only stick with their program, but see better results as well. Social support is key in all areas of life from succeeding in fitness to combating against depression and a negative mood.

Likewise, on the workout front, if you know that they're going to be there bright and early, depending on you to show up, when that 6 AM buzzer sounds to wake you up, you'll be less likely to slam the snooze button and go back to sleep and more likely to get yourself out of bed and show up so that you don't disappoint them.

Furthermore, by making your workouts a bit more of a social affair, this too can help to improve your desire and tendency to stick with them as well.

Most people do tend to be quite social by nature, so if you're having others join you in your sessions, this will go a long way towards keeping you committed to the program plan. You'll enjoy the workouts more, put in more effort, and make better progress going onward.

If you can, try and get a program partner who is at about the same level of you in terms of your overall fitness. This will help ensure you're both doing similar programs (they might even decide to do this one as well and do it right along with you) and that you're both going through similar experiences.

Most often those who are very advanced will want a training partner who is more at their level anyway, so chances are you'll natural pick someone who's more in line with where you're at.

Journaling

The next motivational technique to consider is journaling. Journaling is one of the best things that you can do in a number of instances to help keep yourself going.

First, if you ever reach a point where you strongly feel like you just might toss in the towel due to being so frustrated and angry with some element of your program or the actions you've taken, rather than falling off the bandwagon or rushing to food for comfort, try pulling out that pen and writing in a journal.

We tend to carry our emotions along with us, constantly ruminating over them as they continue to cause us emotional turmoil.

Getting them out on paper however can release these emotions and help you start feeling far better again.

Journaling can be a very freeing experience and while you may feel slightly funny doing it at first, as you keep going and get those emotions out, you will find that you start feeling far better after each session you do.

When you're doing your journaling, you'll want to find somewhere quiet to sit where you won't be disturbed for at least 5-10 minutes.

Then, write down in that journal, not stopping for the entire time duration that you've set.

Even if you have to repeat the same sentence over and over again – that's fine just as long as you *keep going.*

That's the key.

While this may sound odd, when you force yourself to keep writing, you may just be surprised at what comes out and down on that paper. Thoughts that you never really realized that you even had may be revealed and then you can go ahead and put some effort to deal with these thoughts and feelings so that they are no longer an issue for you.

For anyone who suffers from emotional eating, where you eat rather uncontrollably even when you aren't hungry, this can be a great way to get past this issue. Until you address those underlying reasons that are driving you to eat, they're going to constantly be playing a factor in your life and the problem will continue.

But, by addressing those reasons, you can avoid this entirely.

Another way that you can use the practice of journaling to keep you motivated is with tracking. We already mentioned this earlier when we talked about the top mistakes that you must avoid, but here again, this is a powerful motivational tool.

When you see the amount of weight that you're lifting going up higher and higher, make no mistake about it, this will definitely serve to motivate you and get you feeling well again.

So don't discount journaling. Find a pen and pad of paper and get to it. Remember that no one is going to see your journal but you, so put whatever you want in it – don't hold back. It's the revealing of all your innermost thoughts, feelings, and emotions in the journal that helps to ensure that you are reaping all the benefits that this motivational technique has to offer.

Finding A Mentor

Moving along, the next motivational strategy that you may want to use yourself is to find a good mentor.

A mentor is someone that you simply look up to – someone that will provide guidance and help ensure that you continually are inspired to achieve more and more yourself.

A mentor can be someone you know in real life, someone who you've met online, or just someone that you have seen in magazines and always like reading their advice and what they have to say.

In the base case scenario, the mentor would be someone who you can converse with on a day to day basis if needed, going to them for advance or help as you require it.

As more and more people go online for help with their workout and nutrition plans, finding a mentor online is becoming far easier and very often you can easily reach out and connect with these people.

In other cases, it may be a personal trainer or someone at your gym who is your mentor, helping you with your own approach when you need it.

Using Your Motivating List Of Reasons

The next motivational strategy to be considering is coming up with a list of reasons why you want to be doing this program in the first place.

We talked about this a little in the goal setting section, but here, you basically want to write down as many valid reasons as to why you are taking steps to become more fit – increasing your activity habits and improving your diet.

What is doing all of this going to give you?

The more reasons you can get down on paper for this, the better this technique is going to work for you.

Try and list both internal as well as external reasons. Internal reasons would be for factors such as improved health, lower risk of disease, more energy, and so on.

External reasons would be reasons that have to do more with appearance – the improvement to your looks for instance or reaching a certain body weight and being able to get into clothing that you want to wear.

If you can get both types of reasons down, this will be the best case scenario because both motivate you in different ways.

Once you have this list of reasons down, you want to be reading that daily, or possibly even more than once a day depending on just how badly you need that motivational boost.

Take some time each morning when you first wake up to read your reasons. This will ensure that they are always fresh in your mind and that you can call them up anytime you need them and are feeling slightly less than motivated to carry on.

In addition to this, any time you feel like you're starting to struggle and are at a risk of falling off the bandwagon, read over those reasons at that point again.

They'll give you an instant jumpstart because you'll be reminded of your ultimate goals once again and why you are moving forward to do the things that you want to be doing.

Remember to update this list frequently if it changes as well. The reasons you're doing the program may change at various points in time and the more valid these reasons are, the more applicable they will be for you.

 Get an Edge!

Consider setting your goals as reminders in your email program so that at various points throughout the day, you are automatically reminded of what it is you're working towards. You'll have sky-high motivation 24/7!

Participating In An Event

The next motivational tip and technique to consider doing is to begin participating in an event of some sort. For instance, you might sign up to run in a 5km road race or decide to compete in a fitness competition (bodybuilding, fitness modeling, and so on).

Having this ultimate goal – a goal that does have a firm dead-line enforced by an actual event can sometimes be just the trick to get you fully motivated and pressing onward.

In addition to this, many people will find that these events are highly enjoyable as well and that may inspire you to continu-ally keep at them, making it something that you're now pas-sionate about and will do from this day forward.

Participating in an event is also a great way to meet other like-minded individuals, so that's something to keep in mind as well. The more often you can surround yourself with other people who are striving to reach similar goals you are and that lead the active and healthy lifestyle, the more likely it will be that you continue to do so as well.

They say that you are the sum of the five people you're closest to, so make sure that those five people are people that you feel you would want to strive to be like.

Taking Progress Pictures

Moving along, the next motivational technique that can be used is taking progress pictures as you go about your journey.

You should be most definitely doing this as doing so will go a long way towards keeping you focused on the end goal and seeing how your hard work has paid off.

It's hard to see changes on a day to day basis that are taking place, but when you look at your body across a period of two weeks or longer, change will definitely be evident.

When you take your progress pictures, aim to take them at the same time each day wearing the same clothing each time as well.

This will help to ensure that you are getting the most accurate representation of the progress you're making since you will not have any outside factors impacting how you look (such as water retention, different forms of clothing and so on).

If you can, your best bet is to also take them first thing in the morning because this is when you will be retaining the lowest amount of water, so you'll be looking your leanest.

As soon as you start eating for the day, depending on what you're eating, that will influence how your body appears.

So taking pictures first thing in your underwear would essentially be the best route to go when it comes to getting the best quality pictures.

 Get an Edge!
Some people, especially women will be very motivated by scheduling a professional photo shoot at the end of 3-6 months as a reward for their hard work. This can make for a romantic gift to give your husband as well if you choose to do a lingerie shoot for the first time since you're now confident in how you look.

Getting Workout Music In Place

The next motivational technique to think about getting into place is finding yourself some new workout music. For many people, this is one of the most beneficial ways to keep themselves motivated and seeing results as they go about their workout sessions.

In some cases, music can be so powerful that you'll find once you start using it, you can't workout without it.

Most people will do best finding workout music that's upbeat and makes them want to get up and dance as this will get their energy levels up during the session and them putting in maximum effort.

Other people may prefer harsher music that helps them get out any anger or tension they might experience, so you'll need to judge your own personality type and what you think may work best for you.

Experiment with a few different variations to see what produces good results and try and change your workout music regularly. There's nothing like a good song to get you pumped up and wanting to keep up the pace of your session.

Another advantage to using workout music is the fact that it will also help to send a message to other people not to bother you.

If you're listening to music, chances are they won't attempt to disrupt you and begin talking to you, which would severely hinder the intensity of your workout.

Chatting between sets and getting distracted is one of the worst things you can do when you're going about your workout as far as your progress is concerned so this helps you overcome that.

Of course if you're working out at home that won't be an issue, but when you're working out in a public, commercial gym, it's often something that you may find yourself dealing with.

Maintaining Sufficient Variety

The next quick tip to remember that will help with your motivational level is that you must be sustaining good workout variety as you go along with the program as well.

This is something that many people overlook as they get stuck in their groove, especially with their diet, eating the same thing over and over again.

Do this and you can rest assured that you will be falling off the bandwagon in no time.

If you're using the workouts that we've provided in this book, you won't have to worry all that much about sufficient workout variety as that will be built right into the program plan.

However on the diet side of things, it's important that you are constantly trying new recipes and switching things around so that you don't become bored.

For instance, you might try preparing a new vegetable you've never eaten before or you might look at converting your classic favorite recipe into a healthier variety.

There are so many different ways that you can improve the nutrition of a given recipe if you just know what you should be looking for.

If you eat the same foods day in and day out, boredom is bound to set in, so taking the steps you need to in order to reduce this from happening must be a top priority.

With so many different recipes out there to choose from, there's no reason that you should be ever eating the same thing for days on end anyway.

Holding A Competition

Finally, the last thing that you might want to consider doing as you get going on your program plan is to hold a little competition amongst you and a few other people who are striving to reach similar goals.

For example, if weight loss is the primary goal for everyone, set a contest to see who can reach their goal the fastest – and have a prize giveaway for whoever achieves it.

For anyone who does tend to have a very competitive spirit, this can be an excellent way to really improve the results that you see and bring out your best efforts.

While there will be a few people who don't react so well to a contest or like set-up, most people will find that this definitely does help to push them along.

So there you have some of the top motivational techniques that you'll want to use and consider as you go about this program plan. If you can pick and choose at least a couple of these and get them into place – alternating between them as time goes on, then you can rest assured that you will be doing everything you can to foster higher motivational levels overall and reduce the chances that once again, you end up falling off the bandwagon.

So now that we've finished talking about how to master your mindset and stay motivated as you get started with the program, it's time to move on and give you the nutritional foundation of knowledge that you need in order to see maximum results.

Part 2

CHAPTER 5:
Diet And Exercise – Why Both Are Required For Optimal Results

Many people who are getting started with their plan to lose weight will wonder if they can't just diet or just workout.

Why must they do both?

While some people are fine simply accepting the fact that they should diet as well as exercise, there are always those who wonder whether they can just exercise and not diet or vice versa.

Perhaps you really love to eat and don't mind exercising, so you think that if you exercise enough, you won't have to watch what you eat. You'll just burn it off in the gym.

Or maybe it's the opposite. You really could take or leave food but exercise – yeah, you hate the gym with a passion. You'd really rather not get sweaty, even if it means eating far less food. To you, that is one trade-off you are most certainly willing to make.

So, can these individuals have their way?

Can you just exercise and not diet?

Or just diet and not exercise?

When it comes to losing weight, while you can just diet and not exercise, your results will not be nearly as good as they would if you had put an exercise program into place.

And as for exercising and not dieting, choose to go this route and you will be climbing a never ending hill to try and reach that goal.

Let's look at why.

The Role Of Diet

First let's talk about why you need to diet. Dieting – or rather – practicing smart nutritional strategies, is what will be necessary to create the calorie deficit in order to get fat loss taking place.

Remember, to lose body weight, you need to consume fewer calories than you burn off over the course of a day. If you don't achieve this, it doesn't really matter what you eat, you won't see results. If someone tries to tell you any different, you know they are not educated in the basic process of weight loss.

It's a simple law of energy.

By creating a negative calorie balance in the body, you force the body to start using its own tissues for fuel sources – with the hope being it turns to body fat.

Now, you may think that you can just exercise more and therefore achieve the same effect.

The problem is that most people do not realize just how much exercise you would have to do to make up for a few small dietary errors.

Let's say you love cheesecake. You can't get enough of it. Day and night, you think about cheesecake (YUM!).

Did you know that most average cheesecakes contain about 600-800 calories per slice?

That is a LOT. Do you know how much exercise it takes to burn that off?

An hour easily – likely more unless you're working so intensely that after that hour, you're about to pass out due to exhaustion.

Make a few small dietary mistakes (okay, you may call them 'indulgences' so you feel better about yourself), and you'll be doing your time at the gym each and every day.

And let's face the facts, most of us simply do not have this amount of time. We're busy and as much as you may love your food, spending two to three hours exercising each day is just not going to happen.

Not to mention the fact that even if you tried to exercise this much, you'd likely get about three or four days into it and end up feeling burnt out, fatigued, and most likely injured. Remember how we talked about the mistake of doing too much exercise earlier? Well, here is why this often happens.

You cannot out-exercise a bad diet, so I would not even recommend trying.

It's just far easier to slash 500 calories per day (which gets you losing one pound per week) from your diet than it is to start exercising to burn calories. While most people don't realize just how many calories are in the foods they are eating, they don't realize how easy it can be in some cases to reduce their intake by 500 calories.

Little things such as omitting the cream from your coffee or swapping out that morning bagel with cream cheese with a slice of toast and some egg whites instead will pretty much do the job for you.

It can be that easy, especially when your diet has lots of room for improvement.

There is another purpose of exercise and we'll look at that next, so don't think that this means you shouldn't exercise.

In addition to creating the calorie deficit required for fat loss to take place, another role of your diet is to improve health.

 Get This!

Those who focus on the health benefits of foods are more likely to make proper food choices than those who focus on the calorie and fat content of foods they shouldn't be eating. Focus on the positive elements of building a good diet rather than the negative elements of avoiding bad foods – you'll do better.

Remember what we said earlier – health should take top priority.

Without health, you have nothing. If you're putting junk into your body, what do you think you're going to get out?

Definitely on a healthy, happy body, that's for sure.

So start putting more attention towards the foods you eat. It is the greatest determinant of success. Diet can easily account for up to 80% of the results you see.

It is that important.

The Role Of Exercise

So now you might be wondering, if diet is so important, what does that mean for exercise? Do you even need to be exercising?

The thing to realize as far as exercise is concerned is that while exercise does burn calories, more importantly, it's going to signal to the body that you need to maintain your lean muscle mass tissue.

If you aren't giving your body the signal that it is going to have to use its lean muscle mass (through performing more intense exercise), you can't expect to sustain your lean muscle mass tissue for long.

In addition to helping preserve your lean muscle mass, another reason why exercising is a must is because doing so is also going to help you boost your metabolic rate for hours after the workout is completed, as long as that workout is structured properly.

This is something that we're going to talk about into much greater detail shortly when we get to the exercise chapters, but if you can structure your workouts in a certain way, you can increase the total number of calories you are burning at rest as you go about the rest of your day for up to 48 hours.

So basically, you'll do your workout and then continue to burn calories faster for up to 48 hours after. This means great things for your overall fat burning capacity as you can imagine.

Essentially, you'll be losing fat faster without having to do more work.

If that's not a win-win for fat loss, I'm not sure what is.

Finally, exercise also has so many health benefits that this cannot be overlooked either.

It'll help with everything from improved muscle and bone strength to increased heart health to lowering your risk of depression.

It's really the cure-all for a number of ailments so when you combine this with a proper diet plan, you can rest assured that you are doing everything you possibly can to become the healthiest you ever.

So hopefully you can now see why diet and exercise are important for fat loss. You really shouldn't have one without the other. They go hand in hand – kind of like peanut butter and jam. While you could have just a peanut butter sandwich, it doesn't quite taste the same.

When both are in place, you will see better results than you ever imagined possible.

Remember that exercise doesn't have to take hours and hours each day, so if you're one of those people who prefers not to exercise because programs you've used in the past required you to put in so much gym time that you didn't have time for much else, this program will be different.

Likewise, you definitely don't have to starve yourself on your diet either, so that problem is going to be out of the equation.

You can eat, enjoy yourself, and feel satisfied – and still lose weight.

We'll be showing you how very shortly.

Getting the combination together isn't all that difficult if you know how to do so effectively.

So now that we've covered why you need both exercise and diet, let's begin our discussion of the concept of calories and why it's so important to you.

Chapter 6:
Everything You Need To Know About Calorie Intake

The content you are about to read is easily going to be the most important part of the book, so read very carefully and thoroughly. This information is not to be taken lightly as it will make or break the results you see.

When it comes to nutrition, the very first step is going to be getting your calories down in proper alignment. Now, when many people hear the term 'calories', their mind instantly does a few flip-flops and dread might set in. Or, perhaps you start thinking about a highly restricted intake and worry that you'll never be able to stick with any diet that takes calories into account.

You don't want to be bound by some number – having it determine whether you succeeded or failed on your diet protocol.

But the fact of the matter is that calories are essentially going to determine which direction your body weight moves.

If you take in more calories than you burn off over the course of the day, you are going to *gain weight*.

If you take in fewer calories than you burn off over the course of the day, you are going to *lose weight*.

If you take in around the same amount of calories as you burn off over the course of the day, you will *maintain your body weight*.

Therefore, if you can get the calorie balance part of the equation down pat, you basically have completely control over which direction your progress moves.

Now, before you start thinking that as long as you reach X number of calories in any given day you are basically assured you'll see success, there are some critical factors to know.

 Get This!

When you overconsume calories on a single occurrence, your rate of oxidation will go up dramatically to prevent fat gain. This is especially the case if you just ate a very high carbohydrate meal.

First, your metabolism will adapt. Take in a very low level of calories each day and you will start burning more to compensate. This is the body's defence mechanism which we talked about earlier that is designed to prevent you from starving to death.

It's very powerful and will make its appearance – make no mistake about that.

The second thing to note is that while calories determine which direction your body *weight* moves, it's your food intake that will determine whether that weight that you're losing is fat mass or lean muscle mass tissue.

If you want to body fat – which must be the priority, then you absolutely must focus on eating the right combination of foods along with only high calorie foods.

Do that and you will see the most optimal results. While you can get smaller just focusing on calories alone, this is not what will assure that you sustain good health all around and make the most of your weight loss program.

It's the combination of the proper calorie intake and the right foods that you need that's essential for success.

In terms of the calorie deficit you're going to use, you want a good calorie deficit, but a reasonable one.

250-500 calories per day will produce a good rate of fat loss, ½ to 1 pound per week, which is where most people should be.

Those who have a high amount of weight to lose (30+ pounds), may be able to take this up a little higher and use a 750 to 1000 calorie deficit, but tread lightly when doing so.

Realize that the leaner you are right now, the faster and harder your body is going to fight you to keep losing weight simply because of the fact that you are closer to starving to death than if you have a high amount of excess fat on your frame.

For those that are leaner however, slow and steady is very much going to win the race nine times out of ten.

You'll feel better as you lose the weight, you'll have a much higher chance of actually maintaining the weight loss that you do see, and you'll also be a whole lot happier as you go about the dieting process as well.

So now that you know why figuring out your calories is so important, let's look at how you pinpoint how many calories you should eat.

Your calorie intake target to get six pack abs is made up of three different components:

- Your BMR
- Your TEF
- Your Activity Level

Let's look at each one of these individually.

Your Basal Metabolic Rate

The very first thing that you need to take into account is your basal metabolic rate. This essentially refers to how many calories your body needs to consume each and every day just to stay alive.

If you were to lie in bed each day without moving a muscle, this is the amount of energy it would take to keep your brain functioning, your heart beating, and your lungs taking in the oxygen they need to keep you alive.

Your basal metabolic rate is fairly determined by your body weight and lean muscle mass, meaning that those who have much more muscle mass tissue will have a higher resting metabolic rate than those that don't.

We mentioned this earlier when we talked about the power of building more lean muscle mass. The more lean muscle mass you can build, the faster your progress is going to go along.

In addition to that, other factors will influence your metabolic rate as well.

These include:

- Your diet

As you'll be seeing shortly, if you structure your diet in a certain manner it can give you a slight boost to your metabolic rate as you'll burn off more calories simply processing your foods. In addition to this, if you avoid those crash diets that so many people go on, this too will help ensure that you're maintaining a higher metabolic rate the entire way through the program.

- Your exercise regime

We'll be going over this one into greater detail as well, but for now note that the more intense exercise you do, the faster your metabolic rate will tend to be. Over exercising, especially doing hours of cardio training tends to have the opposite impact however and will only decrease your metabolic rate further.

- Your sleep habits

One thing that many people completely overlook in their quest to get leaner is the sleep habits that they're using on a day to day basis. If you aren't sleeping as you should, this too will influence how fast you're burning calories as you go about the day and possibly more important, will also influence your likelihood to convert calories you do eat to body fat storage.

- The climate that you live in

While this isn't really something that you can go adjusting, if you live in an area that is much cooler, this can boost your calorie burn. Your body will have to work harder in order to maintain its internal body temperature, therefore increasing your overall daily calorie burn. Shivering itself burns off a very high amount of calories, which indicates the impact that climate can have.

Clearly though, standing in the deep freeze to boost your calorie burn is not a viable fat loss solution, so this element plays little role in day to day calorie burn.

- Metabolic enhancing compounds

Finally, the last thing to note that can boost your metabolic rate up higher is certain metabolic enhancing compounds. This includes things such as the catechins that are found in green tea, caffeine, and capsicum, which is found in cayenne pepper as well as red hot chili peppers. These are a few of the things that you can consume that would theoretically cause your body to burn more calories at rest.

So as you can see, while resting metabolic rate is still relatively constant, there are certain things that can give you an edge here and help you win the war against body fat.

It's impossible to come to a 100% completely accurate estimation of your resting metabolic rate because of all these factors that are in play, so instead we use an average estimation equation and if you have some of these working in your favor – bonus, you'll likely burn up body fat faster than those who don't.

We'll show you the equations that can be used in a second, but right now, let's talk about another factor that gets put into the mix (which these equations account for).

The Thermic Effect Of Food

As we mentioned in the list above, the foods that you're eating can cause you to burn a little more calories each day if you're eating right. This is referred to the thermic effect of food, which measures how many calories your body is going to burn simply breaking down the food you eat. Each and every time you eat a meal, your body is going to burn off calories digesting it, so this gets added to your daily calorie burn.

Different foods will require a different amount of energy to break down and digest.

For example, if you were to eat 100 calories of pure protein, you would burn off about 25 of those calories simply through the digestion process alone.

If you were to eat 100 calories of carbohydrates or dietary fat, this number now changes and you'd only be burning off a measly four and two calories through the process of digestion.

And while 21-23 calories may not seem like that much of a difference, when you're talking about a 1500-2500 calorie intake (which is where most people will be for fat loss to occur depending on their body weight, gender, and activity level), it adds up quickly.

To illustrate this, let's say that you are taking in a fat loss calorie deficit of 2000 calories.

If you take two people, one eating 20% of their diet from protein (200 calories) and another who's taking in 35% of their diet from protein (700 calories), the difference in total calorie burn *simply because of digestion* will be around 125 calories per day (175 calories – 50 calories = 125 calories).

Again, you might think that 125 calories isn't all that much to get excited about, but if you eat in this manner for the course of one month (30 days), you've now burned off an additional 3750 calories, which is a little over one pound of pure body fat.

And you did nothing else but eat more protein. So at the end of the one month time frame, the person who's diet is 35% protein loses one additional pound of body fat compared to the person who's diet is only 20% protein.

Obviously you can take this concept too far. I wouldn't recommend that you go off eating a 100% pure protein diet as that's neither safe or healthy, but it is helpful to know that if you do eat a higher protein diet, your results will move along more quickly than if you didn't.

There's other additional benefits to eating a higher protein diet as well, ones that we won't get into right now, but later on in the macronutrient section that will further illustrate why eating a higher protein diet is a very wise move if your goal is optimal fat burning.

In the equations that we're going to provide you below, the TEF factor (thermic effect of food) is accounted for in the equation already and most are set to around a 15% total daily calorie burn because of digestion, which is about right for those eating an average standard diet.

If you do adopt the higher protein approach we will have you using in this protocol, you should come to see slightly greater levels than this, so once again, you'll be at a slight advantage here.

Your Daily Activity Burn

Finally, the last thing that you must take into account is your daily activity burn. This is essentially going to refer to how many calories you burn off on a day to day basis going about your normal lifestyle activities.

This is the most variable component of all three of them as each and every person will have a wide variety of activity levels. In addition to that, you yourself may be more active on certain days than others, so it's a constantly fluctuating figure.

It would be impossible to again know this value with 100% certainty, so instead you often simply use multiplication factors to estimate this value.

For this section, you'll use the following estimates (each assumes a few workouts per week – if you were an athlete training hard for instance, you would need to bump up your numbers to the next level):

- Sedentary: 1.1 (office job)
- Lightly Active: 1.2 (office job but you're on your feet often throughout the day)
- Moderately: 1.3 (on your feet all day – hair dresser, teacher, store salesman)
- Very Active: 1.4 (constant movement – manual labour, construction worker, etc)

We'll utilize these next when we figure out your target daily calorie intake.

So now that you know the three factors that go into determining how many calories you are burning up on a daily basis, it's time to take a closer look at the formulas that can be used to estimate this.

Get This!
Those who lead active lifestyles and don't go to the gym at all are more likely to maintain their body weight than those who are sedentary apart from their hour-long gym session each day. Lifestyle activity counts!

There are three basic methods that can be used depending on how intricate you want to get. They are:

- The Quick method
- The Harris-Benedict Formula
- The Katch-McArdle Formula

We'll now discuss each of these a little further.

Quick Method formula

This formula is generally used to calculate people's caloric requirements also known as TDEE (total daily energy expenditure), so it'll take into account your BMR, TEF, as well as your Activity Factor. It's the fastest and easiest method (for those of you who hate math with a passion!).

General rules:

Fat loss = 12 -13 calories per pound of bodyweight

Maintenance = 15 -16

Weight gain = 18 – 20

There are a few things to note about this method. First, it doesn't account for body fat. This is vital because methods that do take into account how much body fat you have and how much lean muscle mass is present on your body will always be far more accurate.

So a formula that doesn't take into account body fat percentage may overestimate your total daily calorie requirements for those who have a high body fat percentage and underestimate it for those who are quite lean. Unfortunately, this is exactly opposite of helping you reach your goals.

This is also why some people who are really sedentary and who do have quite a bit of fat to lose will need to use a multiplier of around 10 calories per pound rather than 12-13 to see fat loss taking place.

The second issue with this method is that it doesn't really take into account large fluctuations in activity level but rather just uses a standard value. So if you're either very inactive or very active, it won't be all that reliable for you.

But it is easy, so it has that going for it.

Let's look at the next method.

The Harris-Benedict formula

Using this method is going to much more accurate than using the above quick method, but it's not the most accurate out there (which we'll get to in a second). This method does take into account activity levels much better, but it doesn't account for lean muscle mass, so that element is still missing from the picture.

You will use this method however if you don't know your lean body mass, which many people don't, so it tends to work well for them.

Here is the formula to use.

Women: BMR = 655 + (4.35 x weight in pounds) + (4.7 x height in inches) - (4.7 x age in years)

Men: BMR = 66 + (6.23 x weight in pounds) + (12.7 x height in inches) - (6.8 x age in year)

Since men typically have more lean muscle mass than women do, they will have higher calorie requirements, thus the need for their own equation.

You will need to account for activity level however, and the following will do just that (these are the same values that we mentioned earlier).

- If you are sedentary (little or no exercise) = BMR x 1.2
- If you are lightly active (light exercise/sports 1-3 days/ week) = BMR x 1.375
- If you are moderately active (moderate exercise/sports 3-5 days/week) = BMR x 1.55
- If you are very active (hard exercise/sports 6-7 days a week) = BMR x 1.725
- If you are extra active (very hard exercise/sports & physical job or 2x training) = BMR x 1.9

This will have you approximately how many calories you need to maintain your body weight.

So now let's talk about the last and most accurate way to assess your calorie intake, the Katch-McArdle formula.

<u>The Katch-McArdle Formula</u>

This formula is the superior to the other two because it is the only one that will factor in your body fat levels, giving the most accurate results possible.

If you can get a body fat test taken or use some skin calipers (make sure to get a trained professional to do the test), this will really help out as far as estimation purposes go and ensure that you are eating the right calorie intake for the goals that you have set.

The formula for this approach is:

BMR (men and women) = 370 + (21.6 x lean mass in kg)

Since body fat percentage is taken into account, you will not need different equations for both men and women.

To this formula, you will use the same multipliers as you used above.

- If you are sedentary (little or no exercise) = BMR x 1.2
- If you are lightly active (light exercise/sports 1-3 days/ week) = BMR x 1.375
- If you are moderately active (moderate exercise/sports 3-5 days/week) = BMR x 1.55
- If you are very active (hard exercise/sports 6-7 days a week) = BMR x 1.725
- If you are extra active (very hard exercise/sports & physical job or 2x training) = BMR x 1.9

If you can do this one, use it – it will give you the most reliable results as long as you have used a proper method to get your body fat tested.

So now that you have your *maintenance calorie intake,* remember that we now need to add your calorie deficit.

As noted above, 250-500 calories will tend to work best for most people. If you have a significant amount of weight to lose, you might take it up higher to the 1000 calorie mark, but for most people this would be too much. Remember that there are 3500 calories in one pound of body fat, so using a deficit of 500 calories would result in one pound of fat lost per week – which is a good place for most people to be.

Remember that women should avoid ever going below 1200 calories per day and men should aim to stay at around 1500 calories or over per day for basic health needs.

Going lower than this could cause you to risk malnutrition and that is something that we clearly don't want.

So you'll take the number that you arrived at above (using whichever formula you preferred) and now subtract the deficit from it.

This is your new target calorie intake.

It may feel overwhelming, but walk through the calculations, picking whichever method is going to work best for you.

If you do this right, it will make all the difference in your fat loss results, so it's not something that you want to take lightly.

Do it right from the start or all the hard work you put in may be for nothing.

Once you have these calculations in place, don't feel overly stressed out about the process of tracking your calories either.

There are so many different phone applications, websites, and so on that are aimed to help make things easier for you that there's no real reason you should struggle with this.

Furthermore, once you learn the proper portion sizes of food and about how many calories are in the foods that you're eating, the calorie counting will almost take care of itself.

So now that you have the most important element out of the way, let's move onwards and go over what you need to know about the three main macronutrients and how they factor into the equation.

CHAPTER 7:
Taking A Closer Look At The Foods You're Eating

As we noted earlier in the calorie section, if you want to lose body fat, not only will calories count, but the foods that you're eating on a daily basis are also going to factor in significantly.

Furthermore, the foods you eat are going to determine the level of health you maintain, so this is yet another importance reason to be paying attention to your choices rather than just focusing on your straight calorie intake.

When looking at the various foods that you eat on a day to day basis, they can be divided up into three main macronutrients.

'Macronutrients' refers to the different nutrients that make up all the foods that you eat over the course of the day – the proteins, carbohydrates, and dietary fats.

Each of these nutrients plays a different role in the body, so getting the right mix will be important.

If you choose not to regulate your macronutrients, you could suffer from a very uneven distribution, which would then lead you to suffer energy lows, muscle mass loss, nutritional deficiencies, and so on.

Get This!

Each macronutrient has a different role in the body and as soon as you start cutting one out, the body will not function as well as it should. For example, if you cut out all fat from your diet, your body will actually generate fat more easily from carbohydrates than it otherwise would. Balance is key.

Especially when undergoing resistance training, you must be sure you get a good division.

Let's look at each macronutrient on its own so that you can form a complete picture.

Protein

Without question, the single most important macronutrient in the human diet is protein. Protein is absolutely essential for life and without it, in a few short days, you would cease to exist.

The primary role of protein is to form the building blocks in which muscle tissue is made up of. Protein rich foods break down into 'amino acids', which are what is used to repair muscle tissue along with all the other cells in the body.

In addition to this, protein is also going to be utilized to help formulate hormones, neurotransmitters, along with other bodily substances that are required to keep you alive and functioning well.

If you aren't getting enough protein, you will stay in a broken down state for a much longer period of time, never recovering fully before your next workout.

Furthermore, if you aren't taking in enough calories either, you will rapidly begin losing lean muscle mass as your body turns to it as a fuel source.

The sad thing is that for most people, this is the nutrient that does most often go overlooked and that they fall short in.

In addition to providing the building blocks for a wide variety of different body tissues, protein is also going to offer a number of other benefits as well. Some of these include:

Blood Glucose Control

The very first key benefit that protein also offers is better blood glucose control in the body. Adding more protein to your diet is going to help you stabilize your blood glucose better as it'll slow down the release of carbohydrates into the blood, so you don't get that rapid glucose spike followed by crash.

Instead, the glucose is released slowly over time, maintaining your energy level for hours to come after a meal. Of course this will also depend on what types of carbohydrates you eat, but simply adding protein to your meal does tend to provide far better glucose control than if it isn't added.

Hunger Suppression

Next, another key benefit to adding more protein to your diet is that it can help with hunger suppression as well. If you aren't eating enough protein on a day to day basis, chances are you'll be feeling pretty ravenous all day long.

Since carbohydrates do break down so quickly and cause that energy spike followed by crash, you'll be left feeling hungry, weak, and tired after that crash occurs.

The end result is you're driven to consume more simple carbohydrates and the cycle continues on and on. At the end of the day, even despite your higher calorie burn, this could lead to significant weight gain.

Protein rich foods take a long time to break down in the body and digest, therefore adding them to the picture will keep your hunger down and make sure that you can go a few hours at least between snacks and meals.

If you are someone who is concerned with weight loss, this is a very important thing.

Faster Metabolic Rate

Another factor to keep in mind is the fact that protein, as we mentioned earlier, also has the highest thermic effect of food. We discussed this into great detail during the metabolic rate section, so we won't revisit it here.

So how much protein is enough?

The average recommendation for protein for the normal individual not training with workouts is about 0.8-1 gram per pound of body weight. As someone who is heavily involved in training however and who is breaking their muscle tissues down on a regular basis, you may want to take this slightly higher, up to around 1.2 grams per pound of body weight each day.

While this may seem high, keep in mind it is only to be that high while you are on the fat loss diet protocol. Once you're finished losing weight, then you can return back to the lower protein intake set-up of one gram per pound.

Protein rich foods should be consumed at each meal and snack that you eat to help with the balancing of the carbohydrates as we discussed earlier.

When it comes to sources of protein in your diet, you want to choose the leanest meat sources available, along with plenty of fish and seafood, low fat dairy products, eggs, as well as whey protein powder.

All of these are going to provide high calorie protein without the addition of saturated fats or other chemicals or additives.

Summarizing your list of top protein rich foods are:

- Chicken breast
- Turkey breast (white meat)
- Lean steak
- Eggs and egg whites
- Venison
- Fish
- Seafood
- Low fat cottage cheese
- Low fat Greek yogurt
- Skim milk
- Whey protein powder

Making sure to take in a wide variety of different sources of protein is going to be ideal as this is what will ensure you get a good blend of amino acids and nutrients in your diet plan.

 Get an Edge!
Many people are scared of eating too much protein but as long as you are in good health standing, you can safely eat up to 1 gram per day (or slightly more if you are dieting hard). Just be sure to drink extra water when you increase your intake.

Carbohydrates

Moving along, next up we come to carbohydrates. In the standard 'diet world', there is a high amount of controversy over carbohydrate consumption. People everywhere are jumping onto low carb bandwagons because they believe that this nutrient is most likely to lead to fat gain occurring.

Likewise, they firmly believe that carbohydrates are the primary reasons for so many diseases today and if you want to achieve optimal health, they should be cut.

While this is partly true, the key factor some people miss out on is the fact that it's the type of carbohydrates that you're eating more than anything else that's going to matter. Eat the wrong type of carbs and you will be facing weight problems along with health problems. Eat the right types of carbohydrates and you won't have to worry.

The body can only utilize carbohydrates as you go about intense training sessions, so to let yourself fall low on the intake scale would be making a significant mistake.

Your job is to make sure that you time your carbohydrates properly and choose ideal sources. Let's look a bit closer at the various different types of carbohydrates that you'll come across.

Complex Carbohydrates

The very first type of carbohydrate that you must know is the complex carbohydrate. These are the high energy carbohydrates that are complex in structure, meaning they're going to take more time to break down and digest in the body compared to other carbohydrate sources.

As such, when you eat these ones you'll sustain more stable blood glucose levels, meaning you will not experience energy highs and lows that we talked about earlier.

They are higher in calories however due to their complex nature, so you do need to be slightly more careful with the volume that you're consuming.

When selecting complex carbohydrates, the best options are going to be those that are as least processed as possible. The less processing that occurs with them, the healthier they're going to be for the body and the slower they will break down overall.

Good examples of complex carbohydrates to focus on include:

- Oatmeal buckwheat
- Brown rice
- Wild rice
- Quinoa
- Barley
- Millet
- Sweet potatoes and yams
- Bran cereals

If you can focus most of your intake, for the most part, around these sources, you're going to be best off.

Now one additional point that needs to be addressed before we leave this section on complex carbohydrates is the 'whole grain' myth. If you're like most people, you likely see the term 'whole grain' and are conditioned to believe that the food will actually be healthy for you.

But is it really?

Don't be fooled. The fact of the matter is that whole grain is often not much healthier than the straight white food variety that you would have otherwise chosen, so you aren't really going to be that much better off going the whole grain route.

The problem is that whole grain foods are still going to have to go through some degree of processing to get to your lunch or dinner plate. With an apple for instance, you can simply pick that off a tree and eat it.

To get some whole grain bread, a number of steps are going to have to be in place for that bread to get to your sandwich.

While the whole grain varieties of products may not be stripped of their fiber and other nutrients during manufacturing, they are still processed and this does mean they are going to break down more quickly, could contain ingredients that aren't all that healthy for the body, and are going to increase blood glucose levels more than foods that do come straight from the ground.

This increased blood glucose level is also going to cause an increase in blood insulin levels and it's chronically elevated blood insulin levels (due a diet that's high in refined carbohydrates), that leads to belly fat storage.

And further, don't neglect the fact that whole grains do still contain gluten and for some people, this is a big problem because of gluten intolerance.

 Get an Edge!
Those people who consume carbohydrates as part of their regular diet actually see better fat loss results because they are going to be in a more positive mood and more likely to stick with their protocol.

If you are often feeling bloated, suffering from headaches, or having other gastro-intestinal issues after eating foods that do contain wheat, you are going to likely be best off cutting out all of these grains from your diet entirely.

Some people don't have the necessary enzymes to break these foods down and as such, they give their body quite a high level of grief.

So don't be so quick to assume because the food is whole grain, it's a healthy option.

In many cases it's really not.

Simple Carbohydrates

The next type of carbohydrate that you'll come across is simple carbohydrates. These are the carbohydrate varieties that you want to avoid as they are the ones that will lead to that dramatic blood glucose spike followed by crash that we mentioned earlier, plus these are the ones that will cause your insulin levels to shoot sky-high and really accelerate the process of stomach fat accumulation.

Make the mistake of eating these and you might find that you feel as though you're on an energy roller coaster throughout the day.

In addition to that, these carbohydrates are virtually devoid of all nutrition, so are simply not ideal for the body in anyway.

Simple carbohydrate calories also add up incredibly quickly – even faster than most complex carbohydrate sources, so it's a must that you avoid them as much as possible.

Examples of simple carbohydrates include:

- Candy
- Cookies
- Crackers
- Baked goods
- Sugary cereals

- Low-fat ice cream
- White bread
- Rice chips
- Cereal bars
- Bagels
- Packaged snack foods
- Honey/jam

One additional form of simple carb that needs to be mentioned is fruit. Fruit should be thought of as in a different category from the above however as it's going to supply your body with dietary fiber, which is very healthy and will slow down the release of the carbohydrates overall as well, and it will also supply you with a number of important vitamins, minerals, as well as antioxidants.

For this reason, fruit should never be avoided on a healthy eating plan.

The one thing that you do need to keep in mind with fruit however is that it's fruit sugars are half glucose/half fructose and fructose will not be stored in the muscle cells, but rather the liver cells.

This means then that fruits aren't quite as good post-workout in terms of maximizing your recovery since you won't get that muscle glycogen replenishment that you otherwise would.

So try and keep fruits out of the post-run period and place them at other times in the day instead. The one exception to this rule however is the banana, which does have a higher starch component and a lower level of fructose. These can be eaten post-workout and do tend to work great as a recovery fuel source.

Fruits are also lower in calories than many of the other simple carbohydrates listed above, so for this reason they'll also work well for anyone who is being a little more careful about their weight and wants to be sure that they aren't seeing the scale creep upwards.

Fibrous Carbohydrates

Finally, the last type of carbohydrate that you need to know is the fibrous carbohydrate. These are the carbohydrates that are found in vegetables and are also incredibly important to be taking in.

These are very low in calories and carbohydrates overall, so they'll hardly have any influence on your blood glucose levels, so you can eat them essentially without worry. The dietary fiber content they possess will also help ensure you avoid all blood sugar spikes and furthermore, will also help to improve your overall health level by lowering cholesterol, reducing your risk of heart disease, as well as lowering your risk of certain forms of cancers.

Fibrous carbohydrates should be eaten with most meals of the day, however should be avoided right before or after a training session as they are quite bulky in volume and could cause intestinal cramping to occur. Plus, since they don't supply all that much energy overall, they aren't going to fuel you for the coming training that you must complete.

Almost any vegetable is concerned a fibrous carbohydrate, just note that certain vegetables – carrots, peas, corn, and of course potatoes (which are considered a complex carbohydrate as listed above) do contain more carbs and sugars, so you'll want to factor that into your intake.

Now, looking in terms of how many carbohydrates you should be eating on a daily basis, there's no set requirements for carbohydrates, but instead it will vary depending on your target calorie intake for that day and how many dietary fats you consume, which we will talk about next.

Since your protein intake is relatively set and constant, you will adjust your dietary fats and carbohydrates around the protein component.

At bare minimum you should be getting at least 100 grams of carbs per day, assuming no training is taking place, as this is the minimum amount required for the brain to function optimally.

 Get an Edge!

To help make getting your five to ten a day of your fresh vegetables, consider stocking up on pre-cut vegetables or buying them frozen. This makes them far easier to use during meal times and will make sure that you aren't passing them up due to not having enough time during the day to prepare them.

Just keep in mind, for calorie calculation purposes, that proteins and carbohydrates each contain four calories per gram while dietary fats contain nine. Knowing this will ensure you figure out your calculations properly.

Dietary Fats

Finally, the last nutrient that you need to take into account on your program plan is the dietary fat component.

While you may think that cutting out dietary fats is route to go since you want to stay lean, this isn't quite accurate.

In fact, dietary fats are also extremely important for success. The truth is that when you are just going about your day to day activities, you can easily utilize dietary fat as a fuel source and in fact, this is actually preferable because then you will be sparing your glucose stores.

Furthermore, dietary fats have absolutely no influence on blood glucose levels, so they'll help to keep your energy level very stable over time. When combined with a good source of protein, your energy will stay consistent for hours at a time.

Dietary fats also break down incredibly slowly in the body, so will help to control your hunger levels very well also. If you are eating a carbohydrate based diet and keeping your dietary fat intake incredibly low, you will very likely experience hunger on an ongoing basis. In fact, you might find that you're always hungry.

Dietary fat should be kept at no lower than 15-20% of your total calorie intake for a rough guideline. Some people may choose to take it slightly higher than this if they feel they function better on a higher fat/moderate carb approach while others will keep it at this range.

Like with carbohydrates however, it's important that you select your dietary fats properly. Eat the wrong fats and you could set yourself up for numerous health concerns down the road.

You want to be eating primarily unsaturated fats, polyunsaturated fats, and essential fatty acids (or omega fats as they're often called).

These are the fats that will boost heart health, improve your body composition, and help keep your hormone levels normalized in the body, while making sure that you feel your best at all times.

 Get an Edge!
Eating just 5-7 grams of fat with each meal can go a long way towards calming your hunger pains and making it easier to last until your next meal without eating. This is the equivalent of about ½ tbsp. of olive oil or natural peanut butter.

Examples of these fats include:

- Nuts and natural nut butter
- Seeds
- Flaxseeds and flaxseed oil
- Olive oil
- Coconut oil
- Avocado
- Fatty sources of fish

If you can eat these most often and make sure to stay away from unhealthy sources of fats such as saturated and trans fats, which are found in high fat dairy products, processed meats, fattier cuts of meat, and many processed or fast foods, then you will be on your way to maximizing your health while boosting your performance.

So there you have a good idea on the precise foods that should be making up your diet plan. It's vital that you are focusing on smart food selections that will not only nourish your body, but also promote the fat loss process as it takes place.

Rather than simply focusing on reducing your food intake and cutting out as much food as possible, focus on adding healthier foods back into your diet, constructing one that is going to provide the right level of calories and set you up for optimal health.

Now let's talk further about how to go about designing a meal plan that will work to bring you optimal results.

Chapter 8:
How To Make Good Nutrition Work For You

So now that we've talked about the important fundamental concepts of what nutrition is all about, it's time to switch gears slightly and go over more of how you can make all this information work for you.

After all, it does not good to learn about what eating healthy means if you can't actually apply it to your own life.

That's where so many diets go wrong as well – they teach you how to eat healthy but then they don't teach you how to do so in the real world.

If all you did was stay home and never go out so that you could eat controlled meals at controlled times, you'd never falter from your plan.

But we all have lives to lead and therefore, we need to structure our diet in a way that will help us maintain our good eating while still maintaining our desired lifestyle.

So let's look at some factors to consider as you do this.

Being Flexible With Food Choices/Meal Combinations

The very first thing that you'll need to do is learn how to be slightly flexible with your food choices based on what the day brings.

For instance, you might go out to eat at one meal and take in more carbs than you know you should. Perhaps it was a pasta lunch you attended with a co-worker and you know that the bowl of spaghetti you had served up far more carbs than your usual lunch did.

So what now? Is your day ruined?

It doesn't have to be.

All you need to remember is to be flexible with your other meals so that you can easily account for this increased carbo-hydrate intake without it derailing your day.

Cut back on the carbohydrates you eat in the meals that follow and you'll have no problem hitting your daily total targets.

Being able to stay aware throughout the day as you make your various food choices and then simply just cut back when needed will allow you to move through any events you attend, parties you go to, and so on all while keeping your diet intact.

Flexibility is important because not only will it make sticking with your diet easier, but it's also going to help to ensure that you don't get too stressed out by the process overall. Those who get all worked up because they had 20 extra carbs with one of their meals are much more likely to completely toss in the towel on their diet entirely for that day and then really cause some serious damage.

Remember, you are always in control. Should a change in plans occur, you still are in control and can make active and wise decisions going forward.

The minute you 'lose hope' for that day is the minute you invite poor food choices in.

Stay calm, stay focused, and stay in control.

Realizing The Truth About Meal Timing

The next thing to take into account is the truth about meal timing. This is another place where so many people get all worked up and completely lose their ability to stay smart about their protocol.

They've heard that if you eat every three hours during the day – eating mini-meals each time, you will see faster progress because you'll get a boost to your metabolic rate.

Simply put, this is not true.

The first thing to know is that if everything else stays the same – you maintain the same total calorie intake and the same macronutrient distribution (your carbs, proteins, and fats all stay on the same level), it's going to make very little difference if you eat three meals per day or if you eat six meals per day.

The only difference is if you're eating three larger meals per day, you'll get three larger spikes to your metabolic rate.

If you're eating six smaller meals per day, you'll get six smaller spikes to your metabolic rate.

At the end of the day however, it's all going to add up and equate out to the same amount total.

So don't stress out over how many meals you eat. If you prefer eating fewer meals as you're just so busy you don't have time to sit down and eat, so be it – that's perfectly fine.

If you prefer eating more meals as you feel this helps you control your hunger and food cravings better and you keep your energy higher, that's great as well. Learn what's best for you and then structure your diet like that.

Then in addition to that, don't stress at the times you eat either.

I promise, if you go three hours and 20 minutes without eating, your body is not going to start to burn up muscle tissue. You can go six hours without eating and be perfectly fine. You just don't have to eat as frequently as some people believe over the course of the day.

The body is well adapted to go for lengthy periods of time without food and can easily survive that.

This assumes however that your total daily calorie intake is of course in proper alignment. If you aren't eating enough total calories and are missing out on certain nutrients, then it is going to matter if you aren't eating frequently enough because your nutrition needs are going unmet.

 Get This!

Those who consume more calories earlier on the day are more likely to maintain a favorable body composition compared to those who stack more calories in the evening. So aim to eat larger meals first and decrease your food intake as the day goes onward.

Meet your nutrition needs over three meals, four meals, five meals, or ten meals if you really want.

Just remember that as you increase the number of meals you eat each day, you'll also need to decrease the total calories that you're consuming as well in each of those meals so that your total calorie balance lines up as it should. If you go from eating three meals of 500 calories each to six meals of 500 calories each, you can imagine what this is going to do to your overall daily calorie intake.

You'll be rapidly gaining weight if you don't adjust that intake downwards.

So just do be sure to keep in mind that if you choose to eat more frequently, your meal size is going to be much smaller.

Taking Personal Preferences Into Account

Finally, last but not least, you need to take your personal preferences into account. Hopefully I've drilled this through your mind quite readily throughout this guide that personal preferences are VERY important here.

I see far too many diets that completely overlook this. They place people on a plan that has them eating foods that they don't enjoy at all and then you wonder why you can't stick with it.

Well of course you aren't going to be sticking with a plan that has you eating foods you hate – that much is a given.

Likewise, if the plan requires you to eat at certain times that are virtually impossible with your schedule, again, it's just not going to work.

The fact is that weight loss can be achieved in so many different ways along as the foundational elements are in place.

These include a proper calorie intake and sufficient protein.

That's all. The rest is up to you.

Now obviously I'm not saying go load up on candy, chocolate, and pizza and protein shakes while tracking your calories. Clearly that is not going to be ideal.

But if you don't like eating broccoli, don't eat broccoli! If you hate tuna, there are plenty of other healthy protein sources that you can have in your diet instead.

Make choices that you actually enjoy so that this new healthier lifestyle feels good, not like something that you're dying on.

The minute you stop enjoying it is the minute you'll start thinking about coming off of it entirely.

That is when your progress goes out the window.

So there you have the main concepts to know and remember when it comes to making your diet work for you. If you're smart in how you design your diet, it's going to make a significant difference in how well you can stick with it and complete the protocol as planned, so be sure you are not overlooking this factor.

Now let's move forward and talk more about how you can dine out healthfully and still see the weight loss results you want to see.

CHAPTER 9:
Your Guide To Dining Out Healthfully

Now it's time to discuss something that could very easily make or break your diet protocol.

That thing – dining out. Let's face it, life is busy and there are always going to be times when you need to eat in a restaurant or a fast food drive-thru.

Likewise, dinner events will come up and you'll be requested to join others for dinners out so you'll need to know how to eat properly and still maintain your diet.

The scary thing with dining out is that if you do go forward and make a poor food choice, you could easily derail an entire week's worth of dieting. It's not abnormal for a restaurant meal to contain 1000-1500 calories, especially if you are also ordering a drink, an appetizer, and even a dessert (although if dessert is included, you could easily top the charts at 2000 or more calories).

So as you can see, if you're dining out often and making poor food choices, this is a very rapid way to stop all fat loss goals and possibly even see yourself gaining body fat instead.

It's an absolute must that you learn how to make wise choices when dining outside of the home so that you can maintain your diet as best as possible.

In many cases you will be slightly over your allotted calorie intake by a slight amount however as long as you are making smart selections, you can minimize the damage done.

Now, before we move on and talk about what foods you should be eating when you dine in select restaurant locations, it's important to first note that if you do know that you'll be eating out at a given meal, earlier on in the day you should do your best to prepare for this. That way, you can make a bit of extra 'wiggle' room at that meal so that if the calorie intake does go up higher and has you eating over your target amount for that day, you won't have to stress as much since your total target daily intake will still be relatively on track.

For example, let's say you are having a dinner with a friend and you know that you're going to a Mexican place so you will consume a few more calories than your normal meal would contain (Mexican is your absolute favorite).

 Get an Edge!
Always check online before you visit a restaurant to see if they've posted their meals and then use this to help you determine what you'll eat. A little prior planning can help you stick to your healthy eating mission rather than giving into temptation.

If that's the case, then you should reduce your consumption of some of the carbs or dietary fats that you would eat in the meals leading up to that meal so now you can double up at that meal and consume slightly more.

This way, at the end of the day, you're still on par.

This doesn't mean that you should starve yourself however, so make sure that you are keeping that in mind. There's a difference between making some extra wiggle room for yourself and forgoing food so that you're so ravenous by the time you sit down in that restaurant booth you inhale the entire bread basket, a few appetizers, and the largest meal you can find on the menu.

That is not the approach we want you taking here at all.

Instead, you want to be cutting back slightly but still eating the right foods that will keep your hunger down so that you stay in full control when you dine out.

This means forming your earlier meals up out of a lean protein source along with some vegetables for added fiber.

If you choose to eat these meals then when you do go and have your restaurant meal, you'll be satisfied on a smaller portion, thus control your total calorie level even despite the fact that restaurant foods are naturally higher in calories.

So do a bit of prep if you know you're eating out. Of course there are always restaurants where you can choose something that is perfectly healthy and will easily fit on your diet plan so there will be no accommodations needed, but if you know ahead of time you aren't quite sure what's on the menu and healthy food choices may be harder to come by, simply cut back so you're better prepared.

Now that we've covered getting ready, let's equip you with the information you need about what to eat in a wide variety of establishments.

General Guidelines To Follow

Before we get started looking at the types of restaurants individually, it's important that you know some of the general guidelines to follow that will help to ensure that you are making smarter choices.

These should apply across just any restaurant you go to so you can use the at all times.

- Always make sure that you don't consume liquid calories – order water with a lemon or lime. Your body won't register liquid calories like it does food calories so a calorie-containing beverage won't deter you from eating food during the meal

- Never eat from the bread basket. Request it to be removed from the table as soon as you sit down to prevent temptation from hitting

- Consider ordering a half order if it's offered and if not, request that half your meal be boxed up to go instead before it hits the table. It's hard to stop after you're halfway done but if your plate is clean and you ate just half of the meal, you've just practiced instant calorie control

- Avoid desserts and if you must, share with at least one other person

- Always ask for dressing on the side when ordering a salad

- Request the chef go easy on any sauces as this is where calories very often lurk

- Request that any starch side dishes be exchanged for vegetables instead – and request them prepared without butter

- Keep your meat serving size reasonable. There is no reason anyone needs to eat 12 oz. of steak in one sitting

- Avoid any protein that's been breaded – it's the fastest way to ruin an otherwise healthy protein source

- Remove any skin that's on meat that you're served to instantly cut the calories and practice portion control

- If healthy items are available, consider ordering off the appetizer menu rather than the main entrée menu. These are often smaller in serving sizes and could make for a reasonable meal for most people

- Put your fork down between bites to prevent eating too quickly

- Consider going vegetarian for the meal if no healthy meat options are available and be sure to double up on protein when you're at your next meal (at home)

- Check the restaurants website before going to see if their menu and nutritional information is available. This way you go in prepared

- Never be afraid to request for alterations/substitutions to your menu. Doing so can easily save you 200-800 calories per meal depending on what the substitute is

So there you have some quick and simple tips to get you started. Apply these and you'll already be one step ahead of the game.

Let's now move forward and talk about what you should be doing in order to eat as healthy as possible at dine in establishments.

Dine-In Restaurants

When it comes to dine-in restaurants, there are going to be factors working in your favor along with some factors that will be working against you.

Dine-in restaurants are going to offer you the ability to custom-tailor your meal a bit more by requesting those smart substitutions mentioned above. So you do have more control in most cases then when you're ordering take-out or fast food.

That said, what most people would be very surprised to learn is the fact that dine-in restaurant meals can actually contain even more calories than most fast food restaurants.

If you thought your burger and fries meal was a high calories whopper, you haven't seen what dine-in restaurants can dish out. If you aren't watching what you are ordering, you can very quickly and very easily consume upwards of 2000+ calories. All it takes is a few poor food choices.

So on one hand, if you are smart, you can fare very well, but if you're smarter, you can also experience far more damage.

This makes it increasingly important that you do take the following tips into account as you head out to eat at that dine-out establishment.

Let's break the restaurants down by type and give you a few quick tips for each one.

Italian

- Always opt for tomato based pasta sauces over cream sauces

- Choose the smallest serving of pasta possible as most Italian restaurants will serve far more pasta than anyone needs in one sitting

- Make sure that your meal contains a lean source of protein of some variety

- Avoid adding extra Parmesan cheese to your meal at the table

- Avoid dishes that are baked with cheese

- If you see any of the following, avoid: carbonara, parmigiana, lasagna, manicotti, stuffed, frito; instead look for the word 'grilled' – that's your safe zone

- Consider opting for a soup and salad meal with a soup containing chickpeas or any variety of bean to get your protein needs met

- Avoid any bread served with your meal – whether garlic bread or freshly baked bread

- Request that your dish be prepared with very little butter (most Italian restaurants like to load up on butter)

Italian restaurants are often going to present the greatest challenge so you really have to be prepared to deal with these. The dishes are often not only loaded with butter and cheese, both of which really pack in the fat and calories, but they're also going to contain far more pasta – carbs – than anyone needs in a single sitting unless it is a designated cheat or 'refeed' meal.

Go in planning to share a dish with a friend and you'll fare far better.

Mexican

- Always opt for soft tortilla shells versus hard as the hard shells will be deep fried so must be avoided

- Choose real beef strips over ground beef dishes as these will contain less fat and more protein

- Request extra salsa, lettuce, and vegetables and remove the salsa and cheese from the dish

- Consider opting for pinto or black beans over refried beans

- Avoid dishes that contain the following terms: chimi-changa, chalupa, charra, con queso

Using proper portion control will go a long way towards helping to make your Mexican meal more viable on a healthy eating diet plan. Always remember to look closely at the add-ons to whatever meal you're ordering so that you can request certain items such as sour cream and cheese are removed. Guacamole is a good option however as despite the fact it is higher in calories, it's higher in healthy fats so can be a smart move to boost the overall nutrition of your meal and help calm hunger by leaving a higher feeling of satisfaction.

Chinese

- Very often at Chinese restaurants, you will be served larger plates of food to share amongst the people at the table. For instant portion control, order fewer dishes than there are people and you will only be able to eat so much food.

- Never order any deep fried starters, which are very common on Chinese menus.

- Rice is typically the carb source served with these dishes so always opt for steamed (brown if you can) rice over fried rice

- Avoid sweet and sour sauce and use just a small amount of soy sauce instead (be aware however that soy sauce is high in sodium)

- Try and choose vegetable based dishes over rice or meat based dishes for the most part

- Request that any sauce be served on the side

- Go for fish or chicken more often than beef and pork

- Make use of chopsticks – it'll slow you down as you eat so you can practice instant portion control

The big thing to watch out for at Chinese restaurants are deep fried foods along with high sodium foods. These are the main problems that you'll encounter so if you can focus on making sure that you side-step these, you can ensure that you are able to survive a visit to this type of restaurant.

Get an Edge!
Be sure to drink plenty of water if you're going to dine Chinese as this will help ensure that you are not going to feel bloated due to water retention the next day. Chinese food is high in sodium, so practice damage control before you dine in.

Steakhouse

- Choose leaner sources of steak whenever possible and be sure to cut off any visible fat before eating

- Always choose grilled meat rather than fried or breaded

- Opt for a baked potato and request it without butter/sour cream and instead have it with some salsa or diced tomatoes – have this over French fries or mashed potatoes (which are often loaded with butter)

- Choose a side salad with dressing on the side over pasta or rice served with the meal

- Avoid any added cheese to your meal

- If you're going to have an appetizer, opt for shrimp with cocktail sauce or chicken lettuce wraps over deep fried items; raw oysters are also a good choice

- Avoid any type of béarnaise sauce, which is made from egg yolks and melted butter. Instead, look for meat that has been flavored by using pepper or other spices as these will be calorie free

- Opt for grilled fish if ordering fish rather than breaded fish or fish covered in cream sauce

- Opt for a strip steak rather than a rib eye if you want a middle ground cut of beef

The trick at the steakhouse is selecting the right cut of meat and then making sure that the side dishes that it's served with are the lightest options that are available.

French

- Avoid ordering fried appetizers or appetizers of fruit and cheese as these will still be very high in fat and calories; instead opt for raw vegetables, which are labelled crudites or have a salad with the dressing on the size

- Be sure not to eat any of the bread in the bread basket – French restaurants are going to have a wide selection of freshly baked bread so do your best to stay away from this

- A great light meal to choose is a broth based soup, which will be lower in calories and often high in nutrients due to the addition of vegetables

- When ordering fish off the menu, be sure to choose baked, steamed, or grilled rather than pan-fried or baked with butter. Baked fish can either be healthy or very unhealthy, so take some time to learn what's in the fish to make a smart choice

- Stay clear of French fries and order a side salad instead or request a baked potato with salsa

- Always opt for roasted meats and poultry as these will contain fewer calories and be a wiser food choice than those that are cooked in butter/cheese

- Order up Ratatouille, which is a vegetable based casserole dish and can fit into most diet plans

- Choose a fruit based dessert if you need to have something over a higher calorie bread or chocolate based one

When it comes to French dining, if you can learn the menu, you can have success with sticking with your diet. Just be sure to be extra careful about choosing any sort of cheese or butter based dishes as this is the most common problem you'll face when dining in these restaurants.

Pizza Place

- Always order the thinnest crust available as these will contain fewer calories and carbohydrates

- Choose diced chicken if it's available and if not, fresh shrimp; this is far healthier than pepperoni, sausage, or ground beef

- Ask them to go light on the cheese to instantly save calories

- Pile the pizza with as many vegetables as possible

- Limit yourself to just one or two slices – there's no need to eat half a pizza.

Pizza is one of the lesser healthy food choices you can make when dieting as there aren't a lot of truly healthy options. That said, if you choose a smart pizza, you can definitely minimize the dietary damage you do and take in far fewer calories than you otherwise would.

So this wraps up the discussion on dine-in restaurants, now let's move forward and talk more about the take-out/fast food restaurant options.

Take Out/Fast Food Restaurants

When you're on the go, there are going to be those times when you simply want to opt for fast food. You don't have time to prepare a meal at home or may be on the road travelling and it's simply not an option.

Does this have to mean the end of your diet?

It doesn't – as long as you choose wisely. Fast food meals are always going to come with a risk as they typically will be higher in sodium than what you otherwise would eat regardless of what you order, but that said, if you choose wisely, you can definitely practice some good damage control in terms of the total number of calories, fat, and carbs you take in.

Fast food restaurants are notorious for serving up 'super size' options for just a small fraction of the cost of the meal, but you always want to avoid this.

Remember, you may be increasing the total food to dollar value by selecting it but you're also significantly increasing your waistline.

The other entertaining thing that many people do at fast food restaurants that you want to be sure to avoid is ordering up the regular meal – plus a diet soda. Then these individuals think that they are doing their diet justice.

Believe me, you aren't. If you order the wrong entrée, you're just going to be loading your body up with sugar, cholesterol, fat, and calories – all things that will do you harm.

So let's take some time right now to walk you through the main types of fast food restaurants and the healthy choices to be making at each of them.

Burger Joint

- Order grilled chicken over beef as often as possible

- Be very careful about ordering fish as very often it comes breaded or with a high calorie sauce

- Never order breaded chicken – always opt for grilled

- Swap your French fries for a baked potato with salsa instead

- Consider ordering chili if the restaurant offers it

- Always order water – even diet soda isn't your healthiest of options

- If ordering a salad, be sure you get some lean protein with that salad and request that the dressing is one the side. Also ask for it without any crunchy high-fat noodles along with dried fruit or candied nuts. Regular nuts are okay in moderation

- Soup can be a good option if it's on the menu but be sure to opt for the non-creamy varieties

- If you are going to order a beef burger, make absolutely sure it's a single patty and the smallest size available

- Reconsider adding cheese to your burger

- Always be aware of any condiments that get added and consider requesting it without (also pay attention to 'special sauce' additions

- If wraps are on the menu, these can be great choices but be sure that you order one without cheese, mayonnaise, and other high fat ingredients

- Skip dessert – you're already eating fast food so you don't need to add to the problem!

- Consider going bunless – at times, if you're really aiming to watch your calorie and carb count, you should think about opting for a sandwich without the bun. Wrap it in a few lettuce leaves if you prefer.

While burger joints are the most well-known to be unhealthy, they can be not too bad if you make smart choices. Grilled chicken burgers will provide you with a good source of protein and if you pair it with a salad, you'll get some nutrients from the vegetables as well.

Soups and chili's are also terrific selections at fast food restaurants so you'll want to be sure that you are considering those options as well.

 Get an Edge!
Be careful about how much ketchup you use on your burger – it's much higher in sugar than people realize, so not the innocent condiment you may think. Choose relish or mustard instead for a lower calorie and lighter option.

Taco Hut

- Choose a soft taco over a hard taco to cut back on the total fat content of the meal

- Choose chicken over beef whenever possible

- Choose steak strips over beef whenever possible

- Consider black beans – just avoid refried beans

- Ask for your taco to be prepared without cheese or sour cream

- Load up on the diced vegetables along with salsa

- Avocado/guacamole can be eaten in moderation

- Don't order special stacked burritos or tacos – keep it as basic as possible to keep the total calorie count down

- Be sure to drink plenty of water with this meal as it will likely contain far more sodium than you are used to

Taco fast food restaurants aren't typically the healthiest varieties overall as it is harder to make this meal truly nutritious, but you can minimize the damage by choosing the right taco whenever possible.

Practice book portion control by keeping your serving size down and fill up at your next meal instead.

Sandwich Shop

- Opt for whole wheat bread rather than white

- Choose a pita if possible – you can fit more vegetables into a pitta

- Choose thinly sliced bread over thick cut

- Always opt for real chicken over processed if its available

- Be very careful about choosing seafood options as they are often mixed with high fat mayonnaise

- Skip the pepperoni, sausage, or other high fat cuts of beef

- If you must have beef, choose grilled steak strips if available

- Turkey and ham are both viable options if chicken isn't available

- Add plenty of fresh vegetables – as many as possible

- Stay away from cut cheese slices

- Ask for the sandwich to be served without butter or mayonnaise

- Mustard and relish are both perfectly fine condiments

- Pair your sandwich with a salad if you are having a side dish of any sort

- Skip fruit juice/soda and opt for milk or water instead

- Soups can be good options here if available, but be sure to choose non-creamy varieties – broth based should always win out

- Stay away from bagel sandwiches – they're too high in carbs and calories

You can make pretty good decisions at the sandwich shop so this is a very smart place to stop if you are on the go and looking for something to provide you with some energy throughout the day.

While bread isn't the best carb to be eating, when your options are limited, you can make a healthy light meal at this type of restaurant and pick your diet right back up at the next meal.

So there you have your restaurant guide to eating healthy and still enjoying yourself.

Being on a healthy diet doesn't mean you must avoid eating out at all times. While you do want to limit how many times you dine out if at all possible, you still have a life to lead and if you are wise in your decisions you can still maintain your weight loss efforts and be social and satisfy your hunger when it strikes.

CHAPTER 10:
Preventing A Fat Loss Plateau

So now that we've talked about how to eat healthy in the restaurants you go to, it's time to move onto another very large issue that almost everyone will face at some point or another, the fat loss plateau.

The fat loss plateau may just be one of the most frustrating times for anyone on an intense diet or workout program. Things are going along great – you're seeing optimal results and then suddenly it just seems as results come to a complete halt.

What gives?

How come you're no longer making the progress you were hoping for? You haven't changed anything you've been doing, so has your body just stopped working?

Not in the least.

What's going on is that you've now hit the fat loss plateau.

There are a number of reasons why a plateau may occur, so it's up to you to evaluate the situation so that you can come to see which reason is impacting you and what you can do moving forward to change it.

The last thing you want to do is give up hope and just accept that you may not be cut out to lose weight.

That isn't the case at all. If you take the right action steps, you can easily get back on track to seeing results.

Let's look at what possible factors might be at work.

You're Not Tracking Accurately

The very first reason you may not be seeing the fat loss results you wanted is if you're not tracking properly. Remember, you must account for everything you eat and you should be weighing and measuring your foods.

Even small slip-ups in measurement could cause very disastrous results as far as your ability to maintain the proper calorie intake go.

For instance, say you were supposed to have 1 tbsp. of peanut butter twice per day but instead you consumed 1 ½ tablespoons (which is an easy mistake by anyone's account), this now means that you are over by about 100 calories that day.

Do this every day for one month and that is one pound of total body fat that you did not lose because you were making that error.

If you make three or four errors like this, it could completely wipe out the progress that you were seeing, so you must make sure that you are being careful here.

Getting lazy with serving sizes could be the reason you aren't seeing the fat loss progress that you want to be seeing.

 Get an Edge!
The absolute best way to be sure of how many calories you're eating is to get a digital food scale. These don't cost all that much and might just be the most helpful kitchen tool you could use.

<u>You're Not Accounting Properly</u>

The second reason you may not be seeing the success you're after is if you're not account for how much food you're eating.

Are you eating a little bite here and there and not really paying attention to it?

It doesn't matter…you think.

Only it does.

Too many of these little bites can easily add up to almost a full meal, so this could really hinder your ability to lose weight as well.

Track *everything*.

If it goes past your lips, it gets accounted for.

People get lazy with this as well and that can quickly derail progress entirely.

<u>You Haven't Re-Adjusted Your Calorie Requirements After Weight Loss</u>

The next reason you may not be losing weight as you had hoped you would is if you've lost a significant amount of weight and haven't re-calculated your target calorie intake once again. Always remember that if you lose weight, your resting metabolic rate will go down since you now have less total body weight to support.

Therefore, if you've lost 20 pounds or so, your new calorie intake may be your old fat loss calorie intake so you're just maintaining your weight now.

You need to decrease your calorie intake once again at this new lower weight to ensure that you are continually creating that deficit that will have you burning up more body fat as time goes on.

It's a smart move to re-calculate your target calorie intake every 10-15 pounds you lose to ensure you stay on the mark and are constantly seeing progress occur.

Your Metabolism Is Sluggish

Finally, the last and one of the most common reasons why fat loss may come to a slow is because your metabolism is shutting down.

This is due to the hormone Leptin that we've mentioned and the fact that your body has now clued into just what is going on and is saying, 'I don't think so!' It's doing what it can to prevent further fat loss from taking place.

Always remember, your body is on a mission to keep you alive, not necessarily look as lean as you'd like to look.

Therefore, when you are dieting for an extensive amount of time, it's going to be doing what it can to ensure that you are keeping your metabolic rate high at all times and preventing this slow-down from taking place.

The way to do this is to have periodic and regular refeeds or cheat meals (depending on how you want to work this) so that you can trick your body into thinking that it's come off the diet and can start burning up more calories once again.

Basically, if you feed it a much higher level of calories for a good few days, this will help to restore many of the hormones that are associated with your body weight as well as your overall well-being and help to keep you moving along without a problem.

Far too many people get caught up in thinking that if they just keep pushing onwards and sticking with their diet long enough that will be sufficient to see ongoing results but that isn't the case at all.

You must give yourself a break from time to time if you want to avoid the plateau. Don't think of it as taking a step back but rather, taking two steps forward.

You will come back to the diet after the brief break burning up calories at a much faster pace, thus prompting fat loss to occur far faster than you were experiencing beforehand.

There are two ways that you can take this break – either using a 'refeed' or a cheat meal. Both are quite similar but with some key differences to know.

Let's have a look.

Refeed

The reefed is a very structured way of boosting your metabolism so that you burn up body fat faster than before. With the reefed, you are essentially going to be planning to overeat, consuming primarily carbohydrates while keeping the fat content of the diet very low.

The thing to know and remember here is that carbohydrates are going to have the most significant influence on your metabolic rate so they are the ones that you need to be adjusting the most when it comes to boosting things upwards and avoiding that plateau.

Carbohydrate intake is closely connected to leptin and leptin is the primary hormone that will cause hunger to set in, your metabolism to slow, and so on.

Restore leptin and it will go a long way towards helping you get past the plateau. Dietary fat has very little influence on leptin or these hormones however, so by keeping fat much lower on the reefed and really piling in the carbohydrates, you will help to avoid excess fat gain due to too many calories as well as the fact that you are taking in both a high consumption of carbs and fat at once.

That's never really a wise plan if the goal is to keep as lean as you can. You do want this period to be higher in calories, make no doubt about that, but it should not be higher in both carb and fat calories – just carbohydrate calories alone.

Refeeds can last anywhere from five hours to three days depending on how long you've been dieting and how lean you are.

Generally speaking, the more intense and low calorie the diet is and the more strict you have been with yourself, the more often you are going to need to have these refeeds. If you're bringing your calorie intake very low, this means your body will be running scared and shutting down its calorie burning accordingly.

Likewise, the leaner you become as you go about your diet plan, the more likely it is the body starts the metabolic adaptation process sooner because of the fact it's easier for you to get to a point of starvation.

Obviously the less fat you have on your body to provide fuel during times of very low calorie intakes, the more the body is going to fight to give up what fuel it has left.

So for very overweight individuals, the need to reefed will occur much less regularly than those who are approaching single digit body fat levels (or low teens for women).

When refeeding, choose foods that are high in starch carbohydrates while you try and limit the amount of fructose that you consume (in the form of high fructose corn syrup or high quantities of fruit). Some fruit is okay, but keep it to one or two pieces and stay away from the corn syrup.

The reason why you are avoiding fructose during this time is because of the fact that it won't get stored in the muscle cells but rather get shuttled off to the liver where it will be converted into glycogen (at a storage capacity of just 50 grams) and then any further taken in converted to body fat.

So all in all, if you're eating too much fructose, you will gain fat very quickly while if you eat primarily starch/glucose, you'll restore muscle glycogen levels and jumpstart your hormones and metabolic rate as we wish.

Keep fat as low as possible and your protein intake where it normally is. Your protein needs won't change for this day as they pretty much stay constant at all times regardless of what you're doing (if anything, they go up as your calories go down).

So there you have the primary factors to know and consider about a reefed.

Now let's move onwards and talk about what a cheat meal entails.

 Get an Edge!

When you have a reefed, drink some water to keep thirst at bay but don't overdo it if you want to limit the amount of temporary weight you gain. When you eat a high amount of carbohydrates, it's very probable that you will store excess water in the muscle tissue cells as glycogen is formed, so keeping your water intake more reasonable will help you get around this issue.

Cheat Meal

Now we move over to the cheat meal. The cheat meal is quite similar to the reefed with one key difference, anything goes.

While with the reefed, you are going to be strictly limited to those higher carbohydrate foods as we mentioned that are low in fat, with the cheat meal, you will indulge to your heart's content.

There aren't going to be any major rules or regulations guiding the cheat meal. You can basically eat whatever it is that you are craving, not worry about your calorie intake, and just enjoy yourself while experiencing a solid metabolic boost.

This cheat meal will be advantageous since it's very good for providing any psychological relief/stress you're experiencing due to cutting the calories from your diet. If you've been on the diet for a lengthy period of time, chances are very good that you are starting to experience a strong desire to eat the foods that you've cut out and a cheat meal can make doing this permissible.

You will still get some metabolic enhancing effects because even simply taking in more calories during that cheat meal does help to provide a nice boost and let your body know that the diet is over (when really, you plan to go back on it shortly).

That said, because the cheat meal isn't regulated which means you may take in more fat when you have it, this can cause you to start converting more of those calories into excess body fat as well.

So there are pros and cons.

Pro – you get psychological relief very well.

Con – you may struggle with some fat gain if you aren't careful.

It's up to you to weigh the pros against the cons and decide which route to go. If you're someone who naturally craves low fat, high carb food such as pasta, rice, cereal, and so on, then you likely can basically get your 'cheat' meal in by doing a reefed because those are the foods you typically want.

But if you're someone who naturally craves high fat foods, you may not find that the reefed is sufficient to calm your cravings, thus you may still struggle to stick with the diet long term.

Also note that cheat meals are typically done for just one meal or one day, whereas refeeds can last three days at a time.

So that's another difference as well. Some people may choose to combine them, say have a cheat meal once per week and implement a three day reefed once a month as they go on their diet. That can work well to give you the best of both worlds.

So think about what's most important to you here and then choose to structure your diet and cheat/reefed meals accordingly.

One final thing that must be mentioned is that in extreme cases if you've been dieting for months on end without either of these, then sometimes a full blown diet break is required. A diet break is basically that – getting off the diet and just eating at maintenance for a longer period of time.

These will usually last anywhere from one week to a few months depending on your goals and the level of metabolic damage that you've suffered while going about your diet protocol.

The diet break doesn't have to have you eating very high calorie or high carb foods, but rather you just need to be providing enough calories that your body can function optimally (so at maintenance level) and making sure that your carbohydrate intake is at least 150 grams per day.

This is a minimum amount required for your hormones to optimize themselves and for your metabolic rate to return back to normal.

You should be focusing on eating healthy during this period as well because it is a longer duration process so you want to make sure all your nutritional bases are covered.

So there you have the primary information to know about refeeds, cheat meals and diet breaks along with what you can do to get past the fat loss plateau.

There's absolutely no question that it is one of the most frustrating and trying times for anyone aiming to lose weight, but if you keep your cool and just implement one of the above techniques, you can push past it and start moving back on track towards the success you were hoping for.

So this now wraps up the discussion on the theory of dieting. Now let's move forward and talk more about the exercise component of things.

CHAPTER 11:
A Closer Look Into The Exercise Varieties

Now that we've finished with all our discussion on nutrition, it's time for us to switch gears entirely and turn the focus over to exercise.

As we mentioned earlier, while your diet is the most pivotal element that will establish how likely you are to succeed with your fat loss efforts, beyond diet, you must be doing some smart exercise training as well.

Exercise training will boost your health, enhance your metabolic rate, and ensure that you maintain your lean muscle mass tissue.

All musts for success.

This said, not all exercise is created equally. If you choose the wrong types of exercise, you'll be wasting your time.

If you choose the right types of exercise however, you will be moving along, seeing a fitter, leaner, and more firm you taking place.

Gravitating to hours of cardio training however is not the route to take if you want to build yourself a dream body, so this is something that must be avoided.

Many people simply don't fully understand the different types of exercise variations that can be done, which is why they tend to just turn to doing cardio training instead.

If you take the time to get fully educated however, you can come to see why all those hours of cardio training will not be what you're after and why you must change things around and go about the program differently if you're going to see optimal success.

So let's take some time right now to go over the most common forms of exercise so that you can see the pros/cons to each and how they will fit in with your overall program plan.

 Get This!

Those who perform more intense exercise can usually exercise for half the amount of someone who exercises at a moderate intensity and burn up to twice the amount of body fat. When it comes to the game of fat loss, intense exercise wins out almost every time.

Steady State Cardio Training

The first type of cardio training to talk about is your steady state cardio training, which is what we just mentioned. This is basically cardio training that is done on your chosen piece of cardio equipment, be that the bike, the elliptical, or the treadmill.

You'll pick your mode and go at it, working at a moderate intensity level for anywhere around 20-60 minutes. For most of those who are more intensely focused on their weight loss goals, they usually choose the 60 minute mark, doing at least one session per day, seven days of the week.

Bad move.

First, this form of cardio training is doing very little for your fitness level. Sure, it is getting your heart rate up slightly and keeping it there so you will reap a few heart-health benefits from it, but is it challenging your fitness level to move to new heights?

Is it improving your speed, power, and muscular strength?

Is it causing your metabolic rate to increase?

No, no, and definitely not! (if anything, this form of exercise will slow your metabolic rate down as it'll cause you to lose lean muscle mass if you recall from our mistakes discussion).

This form of cardio basically just wastes time. If you truly enjoy endurance related training, then fine, you may just find you get great satisfaction from these workouts and don't especially care if it's not ideal for results. There is something to be said for doing workouts that you do fully enjoy. If you attempt to put yourself on a workout that you hate, it doesn't matter if it's the best type of exercise for you to be doing, the chances that you see results will still be slim because you won't be *doing* that workout session.

You need a workout that you'll actually do and if endurance training is your thing, then endurance training is your thing. But, if you are most interested in maximizing the results that you get from the time you invest in your training workouts, then moving away from endurance training needs to be your priority.

Furthermore, for about 99.9% of the population, you're counting down the minutes until your cardio time is done so enjoyment isn't exactly the word you'd choose to describe these sessions.

You'd say they're more along the lines of torture – and not something that you want to be doing if you're downright honest about it.

Fortunately, you don't have to.

Now, before we leave off on this form of training, there are a few points to note. There will be some instances where this form of cardio training will actually be the best thing for you to be doing.

Those instances?

First, for the very beginner.

If you're someone who has never done any form of formal exercise before, chances are if you dive into things and start doing interval training, you are going to be feeling mighty overwhelmed with it all. You'll wind up pushing your body too hard and believe me when I say it will rebel – with full force.

You need to start by building up a foundation of fitness and often, steady state cardio is the way to do this.

You don't need to be doing hours and hours of steady state cardio however – a few sessions each week will be more than enough and you must also be doing your resistance training activity as well.

If you aren't resistance training, you're making a bit mistake (more on this shortly).

The second instance where you may want to be performing some steady state cardio training is if you're someone who doesn't have the greatest of recovery abilities (you tend to take a longer time to fully recover from intense workouts that you're doing) and you are in the gym doing hard resistance workouts four days per week.

In that instance, you would want to be doing some steady state cardio training. Low to moderate intensity resistance training is going to be far less stressful on the body compared to intense sprint training (which we'll cover next), so by doing this form of training, you ensure that your central nervous system doesn't become overtrained, which would seriously hinder your progress, not to mention make you feel very unwell also.

The body can only handle so much intense exercise each week so if you're really overdoing things, so there must be some balance.

If you can't perform the sprint training for these reasons, then the moderate intensity, steady state cardio training will help you get some cardio training in while making sure that you still feel well overall.

So while it is definitely not the most effective form of workout you can be doing, in some situations, it is the best choice of workout to be doing given the other exercise you are completing.

Just keep that in mind – it's not completely detrimental when added wisely. This means a few 20-30 minute sessions however, not 6-8 hours of steady state cardio per week.

Interval/Sprint Training

Enter sprint/interval training. As far as cardio training is concerned, this is the far more effective method of training that you should be focused on. This is the method of cardio training that will get you results and it's also the method that most people are going to find a whole heck of a lot more enjoyable as well.

This said, it's also far more intense, which can be off-putting to some people, so you need to be prepared to work hard. But if you do, you will be rewarded.

The interval/sprint training cardio protocol is going to have you alternating between all out bursts of very intense exercise with active periods of rest.

So for instance, you'll go as hard as you can for 15-60 seconds and then couple that with an active rest period where you're still moving, but at a very easy pace for about twice as long. This is when your body recovers from the interval you just did.

So you alternate between hard and easy six to ten times to form the complete workout session, starting with a five minute warm-up and ending with a five minute cool-down.

How long you make those intervals will depend on your overall goals. The shorter the interval is, the harder you should essentially be working.

If you're going to do 15 second intervals, you'll be going at about 100% of your maximum effort – basically, full out sprint with everything you've got. As such, the rest periods need to be much longer in relation to that sprint interval.

So for 15 second sprints, you would typically use rest periods of around 45-60 seconds, possibly even longer.

This short duration sprint would be very effective for improving your total level of overall body power and speed capabilities.

As you increase the total duration of your sprint training, so for instance using 30 seconds sprints or 60 second sprints, the intensity will come down some.

Don't get me wrong, you will still be doing very intense sprints, but they won't be as intense as the 15 second ones. You might work at 90-95% of your capability because you have to last longer.

 Get an Edge!
Remember to adjust your intensity of your intervals with relation to how long you are doing them. This ensures that you don't burn out during the session or injure yourself. Both short and longer duration intervals have a place when it comes to achieving a high level of fitness.

At 60 seconds, you'll be focusing more on muscular endurance at top speeds, so note that you will see endurance related benefits from this sprint variety. You typically should never take your sprints beyond the 60 second mark however as that would be moving away from sprint training and more to a moderately-high intensity interval training session.

The best fat burning results are going to come from sprints down up to 60 seconds in duration.

To best help design your sprint training protocol, here are the appropriate rest periods to use with each given interval length.

15 seconds on (sprint): 45-60 seconds off (active rest)
20 seconds on: 60 seconds off
30 seconds on: 60-90 seconds off
45 seconds on: 45-60 seconds off
60 seconds on: 30-60 seconds off

Notice in the last one, if you're really keen on doing a very intense workout that does challenge you from more of an endurance standpoint, you can actually decrease your rest period so it's shorter than your work period.

This would make for a very, very intense protocol however, so note that this is slightly more advanced and you should have a fairly good background of sprint training already in place before moving to such a protocol.

The total number of sprints that you do will again, depending on your fitness level as well as the total time duration that you're doing those sprints for. The longer the sprints are, the fewer of them you will do.

These workout sessions are meant to be short – 15 to 20 minutes (plus your warm-up and cool-down), so you will only have time to get so many in.

If you find that you could keep going past this point and do more sprints still, that's a good sign that you aren't working hard enough throughout the workout session.

While you can choose any mode of exercise to do this workout with, most people will get best results from choosing running or spinning (cycling) as you can accelerate to top speeds quickly with both of these modes.

If you really want a killer sprint cardio workout, then consider uphill running sprints which will definitely test your limits and take your fitness to a whole new level that you've never experienced before (while building the best butt you've ever had as well!).

Hill training is excellent for not only boosting your cardio fitness, but increasing lower body strength as well.

Make sure that you do add that warm-up and cool-down to your sprint training however as otherwise, you'll be at a much greater risk of injury.

This form of training is so intense that if your body is not properly prepared, there is a great likelihood that you may pull a muscle or strain a tendon.

So now that you know what interval training is, what are the benefits to doing it?

Let's go over the primary ones to know.

- Improved resting metabolic rate

Because this training is so very intense, you can expect to see an increased resting metabolic rate for up to 48 hours post-workout. This means you burn fat faster at all points throughout the day, meaning you're going to see a very significant boost to your progress.

This is precisely what also makes this form of training far better for fat loss purposes compared to those steady state sessions. With those sessions, the calorie burning stops when you stop.

- Improved aerobic and anaerobic fitness levels

The next big benefit with this form of training is that it will improve both your aerobic as well as anaerobic fitness levels.

While steady state cardio training will only work you on an aerobic level, this form of training will work you on both, so it's far more effective in that regard.

You'll see greater gains to your overall fitness level by pushing the boundaries and doing more intense sessions.

- Fast and time efficient workout sessions

If you're like most people, you don't have hours and hours in the day to spend doing cardio training. While you may keep up those hour-long steady state sessions for a week or two, after that, your life will get in the way (or boredom will set in, whichever comes first).

The great thing about these workouts, as we mentioned, is the fact that you will be in and out of the gym in less than 30 minutes.

For anyone who leads a very busy lifestyle, this is going to be a huge benefit working in your favor. As a positive trade-off, the more intense you workout while doing these sessions, the shorter they will have to be.

- Decreased resting heart rate

One of the ways that you can monitor your overall health and fitness level is by taking your resting heart rate measurement. Over time, as you perform more and more of these workout sessions, you should come to see your resting heart rate decreasing, indicating health improvements are occurring.

Those who have stronger hearts that are able to pump blood throughout the body more efficiently will naturally have lower resting heart rates because they won't have to be working so hard to get the blood flowing throughout the body.

- Improved heart health

Which brings us to the next benefit these workouts have to offer – improved heart health. By doing these workout sessions, you'll really be working your heart muscle, training it to become stronger over time.

You need to remember that your heart is a muscle as well and requires just as regular of exercise as your other muscles do.

Sprint training is the most effective way to strengthen your heart muscle.

- Increased ability to burn body fat at rest (enhanced fat oxidation)

Finally, the last big benefit that this type of training has to offer is the fact that it will help to boost your ability to burn fat, even while at rest.

Your ability to oxidize fat as a fuel source during rest will go up, so you'll be more likely to be burning up body fat as you go about your day to day activities, rather than burning up glucose/carbohydrates in your system.

This is not only beneficial in terms of promoting greater rates of fat loss, but will also help you maintain higher overall levels of muscle glycogen as well, which means that they will be there when you do need them to perform your intense training sessions.

So as you can see, there is no shortage of advantages to doing interval cardio training. If you're going to do cardio, it is the route to go.

Keep in mind that since it is so intense however, you should never be doing it daily. Two to three times a week will be more than enough to get the results that you're looking for.

Doing it any more frequently than this will just lead you to overtrain yourself, especially if you're doing resistance training, which we'll be discussing next. Some people may choose to just do it once per day depending on their recovery ability and that's fine as well. You need to learn to listen to your body and moderate how much you're doing for optimal results.

Resistance Training

Finally, the last form of exercise to consider is resistance training. Out of all the different exercise variations you could be doing, this is the one that is going to yield the best possible results. This is also the non-cardio mode of training that we'll talk about, however, one thing to note is that if you structure your workouts in a certain manner, you can actually reap cardio benefits from resistance training as well.

So just because it isn't cardio in nature does not mean that you will not see heart-health improvements.

In fact, some people can get away with doing no cardio at all and just focusing on their resistance training workouts instead, especially if they are watching their diet closely enough.

Resistance training is also the mode of training that will best reshape your body, getting you firm, fit, and healthy.

So what is resistance training? Resistance training can take many different forms including lifting dumbbells or barbells, using weight machines at the gym, using resistance tubing bands, or performing basic bodyweight activities.

Basically, as long as you are forcing your body to work against some form of external resistance, you are resistance training.

This said, resistance training with dumbbells or barbells (free weight training) does tend to yield the best results as you'll have the highest possible external load and you'll also be working your core muscles to a larger degree as well.

Whenever you are doing free weight training, your core muscles are going to have to be sitting up and contracting as hard as possible in order to keep the body stabilized, and this means greater overall core strength developments for you.

Since many people do have the goal to get flat abs in their program plan, this clearly is a huge advantage.

Let's take a closer look now at some of the primary benefits that resistance training has to offer.

 Get This!

An effective resistance training workout only needs to take about 60-90 minutes per week, so get past the thinking that you will have to spend hours each week in the gym to see results. That's simply not the case at all.

- Improved Muscle And Bone Strength

The first big benefit you'll get from resistance training is improved muscle and bone strength. By performing strength training, you'll see your muscles getting stronger, which occurs when you break them down after pushing them hard with a stress load they haven't encountered before, and then follow that up by backing off and letting them recover.

In addition to that, since you'll be placing a high external load on the bones, this will cause remodelling to occur and that will also help your bones grow back stronger than they were before, increasing their density and reducing the chances of stress fractures down the road.

This is very important, especially for women as they grow older, as the risk of experiencing osteoporosis is going to be increasing. If you aren't regularly doing weight bearing activities, you will notice a decline in your bone and muscle strength levels and resistance training is one of the best ways to fend off this decline. It is, after all, going to be the most weight bearing activity out there, so offers top notch protection.

- Accelerated Resting Metabolic Rate

Next, one of the most powerful benefits of strength training and perhaps the primary reason why you should be doing this mode of training more often is because it will significantly boost your metabolic rate for hours after the workout is completed.

We talked about how sprint training will increase your overall metabolic rate, but weight training takes this to a whole new level.

With a good strength training workout session, you'll be burning more calories for up to 48 hours after the workout is completed, meaning you'll be torching body fat all day long, just as you were with the sprint training we mentioned earlier.

What's more however and what makes weight training unique is that if you are able to build more lean muscle mass with your strength training workouts, this means that you will actually experience a permanent increase in your resting metabolic rate since you have more total lean mass to support.

Muscle tissue is very metabolically active, so the more of it you have, the more calories you burn doing nothing at all. This is one reason why men don't seem to gain fat as easily as women. They have more muscle on their body so they have a protective element working for them.

You too can get this protective element if you focus on building lean muscle mass. So there are two ways in which you can boost your metabolic rate with strength training compared to the one way in which it tends to occur with sprint training.

For seeing greater rates of fat loss success right now, as well as improving your ability to maintain your body weight and fend off any future weight gain down the road, you simply cannot beat strength training.

- Improved Functional Fitness Level

The next big benefit of resistance training to note is that it will also help to improve your functional fitness level. What do we mean by this?

Basically, by doing your regular workout sessions, you'll see transfer over benefits to your everyday life so that you're stronger than you were before.

Everyday tasks – walking up stairs, carrying groceries into the house, doing anything that involves muscular strength, will now be easier because you have strengthened the muscles involved in performing all of those movement patterns.

Of course this does assume that you are using the right workout program, so do keep that in mind. If you don't form your workout properly, it won't be very functional at all so you may not see these benefits. We'll show you how to ensure that it is so that you reap these benefits.

As you grow older, this will become more and more important as well as the greater level of functional fitness you attain, the higher quality of life you will lead.

One of the biggest issues that many people experience as they grow older is a loss in their ability to perform some of the activities that they formerly enjoyed, so getting on a proper strength training program ensures you eliminate this problem entirely.

- Improved Muscle Tone And Development

Next, another critical benefit to know regarding strength training is the fact that you will see increased muscle tone and development occurring.

This is the primary reason many people do get involved with a strength training program in the first place – by doing so you can see improved body composition and appearance.

If you perform the right combination of exercises, you can more definition to selected areas of your body that you especially want to focus on and target, so if you have a particular trouble spot you really want to be working, resistance training will allow you to hit that exact place.

Keep in mind however that you will never 'spot reduce'. Some people think that by performing enough of an exercise for that area of the body, they can actually cause it to look leaner, but if you have a thick layer of body fat covering that area, this will never be the case.

You need to be reducing fat *and working that muscle group* in order to see the results that you're going for. The combination effect if what gets you more defined. But on the flip side, without that strength training in place, chances are even if you lost weight, you wouldn't get the definition you're after either if there was not sufficient amounts of muscle present to achieve this.

With cardio training, you become a smaller version of your current self. With resistance training, you become a brand new you.

Which do you want?

 Get This!

The heavier weights you lift (within reason – proper form must be maintained at all times), the more muscle tone and definition you are going to see. Do not be afraid to lift heavy. It's your fast track to improved progression.

- Improved Self-Confidence

As you start making positive changes to your appearance, your self-confidence is also going to go up. This is normal and natural and for most people makes sense. The better you feel your body looks and the happier you are with your appearance, the more self-confidence you're going to have.

This said, the positive appearance you're building isn't the only place where your self-confidence is going to get a boost.

In addition to that, you'll also notice that you start becoming more self-confident when you realize just how strong you're becoming and see yourself reaching workout goals that you set for yourself.

Now, your body may take on new meaning.

You no longer view your thighs as 'thick and flabby', as many women do or the men out there may not see themselves as 'scrawny and weak', if that is the case for you.

Now you'll see your body for what it can help you achieve. Maybe you can squat 150 pounds and feel very proud of that fact. Or, maybe they helped you climb partway up a mountain on your last hiking trip.

Whatever the case, your body now is more than something that you view for appearance's sake only. It's now something that serves a purpose – that you know can perform various feats that you put your mind to.

For many people, this is incredibly empowering and helps them build a much better relationship overall with their body.

If you suffer from bad body image issues, strength training is often the form of exercise that can help you get past this.

- Improved insulin sensitivity

Moving along, the next thing that resistance training will help out with is improved insulin sensitivity. This refers to the fact that your body will become more sensitive to the hormone insulin, which means you will be better at managing any carbohydrates you consume.

Those who have poor insulin sensitivity will have to work harder to control their blood sugar after consuming carbohydrates and will also have a greater chance of converting carbohydrates they consume into body fat stores as well.

What's more is that if your body becomes very insulin resistant, this means that you may actually be putting yourself at a serious risk of diabetes.

Diabetes is essentially a condition that comes on due to lack of insulin sensitivity and it's so bad that now it's at the point that your body's cells have stopped responding to insulin altogether.

Strength training is a very good way to prevent the onset of diabetes, and this is critical to note because diabetes is currently one of the more prevalent conditions that is on the rise in our society.

If you use the diet protocol described in this book however along with a good resistance training program, you will be doing everything you can to prevent diabetes from occurring.

- Lower Stress Levels

Finally, the last big benefit that resistance training has to offer is a much lower level of stress as well. Stress is something that you must be taking control over in your life as it can really come back to impact you in many negative ways if you aren't careful.

Stress is something that can be unavoidable at times, but with the right strategies in place, you can help to at the very least, reduce your level. Resistance training is one such strategy.

When you perform intense exercise such as resistance training, you'll be releasing a number of positive endorphins in the body that will give you a rush of energy, cause you to feel good, and help you feel more calm, collected, and relaxed.

Basically, it's like a feel good sensation – a euphoria almost. Not to mention the fact that lifting weight simply proves to be stress releasing in itself as it has a similar impact on the mind as say punching a wall (for those of you who like to use force to release pent up stress!).

So resistance training is one of the healthier ways that you can take out some of your built up anger and frustration.

As you can see, there is definitely no shortage of benefits to be had from resistance training. This isn't even the full list – but it's the main points that will serve to open your eyes best as to why you must be doing this variation of training.

If you can only do one type of exercise variation, resistance training should be your choice.

Of course there are other variations of exercise – group fitness classes, yoga, pilates, etc, and those are fine to do in addition to your program if you wish, but keep in mind that these are the three primary exercise forms that most activity will fall into.

Now before we move forward, I want to take a little bit of time to talk about how your body type will influence the type of exercise you should be doing as this is critical to note if you are to design a workout program that is properly formulated for your body.

How Body Type Will Influence Things

We already mentioned how not every form of exercise is created equally. Well, in addition to that, not every body will respond in the same way to a given exercise program.

Each person is unique in what their body will respond to and if you aren't matching an appropriate workout protocol to your body type, you may be in for problems ahead.

When looking at body types, there are three main types to know: endomorphs, ectomorphs, and mesomorphs.

Let's look at each individually and what this means for your plan of attack.

Endomorphs

First let's begin our discussion with the endomorph body type. If you have this body type, you are likely reading this desperate to find the solution to your weight loss woes.

These types of individuals tend to have a very easy time packing on more body fat and have a very difficult time getting lean. It's almost like their body is out to get them.

They tend to be relatively average height with a thicker build and unlike mesomorphs, which we'll talk about in a second, their 'thicker build' is not due to muscle mass.

These individuals also tend to suffer from a slower and sluggish metabolic rate and may find that they gain fat very readily on higher carb diets, thus going with a lower carbohydrate approach generally tends to yield the best results for them.

These individuals will also typically have to do a little more cardio training as well to get the fat off they want to lose and should focus on being more active in day to day life as well to boost their overall calorie burn and make up for their slow and sluggish metabolic rate.

Furthermore, they may need to use a lower overall calorie intake for all body weight goals (be it fat loss, maintenance, or muscle building) as they just don't have the calorie expenditure that other individuals do.

 Get an Edge!

Remember that you cannot change your body type, so rather than being depressed about your natural tendencies, simply accept them and make sure that you come up with a program plan that is designed to work with your body rather than against it. If you choose the right program, you can still see remarkable levels of progress.

So summarizing their training and nutrition needs you have:

- More cardio training
- A lower calorie intake
- Lower carb diet set-up
- Focus on weight lifting to build more lean muscle mass activity
- Greater daily activity to make up for slow metabolic rate

Ectomorphs

The next body type to address is the ectomorph. As much as the endomorphs may feel like they'd give their left leg to be more like the ectomorphs, if you're an ectomorph, you likely think the opposite.

For you, being of this body type feels defeating because no matter what you seem to do, you stay skinny. Often known as the 'skinny guys' for men or the girls who look like a tomboy, the ectomorph body type is one that's more straight up and down, lacking curves and muscle definition.

Those who have this body type have lightening fast metabolic rates that seem to just speed right up as more food is being fed.

So despite your best efforts to eat more calories with your diet, your body just burns those up as energy, showing no change in body weight.

In fact, for you, it may be just a challenge to avoid losing weight. You eat and eat and yet, you don't gain an ounce.

These individuals, despite all their frustration, can still see results if they go about it in the proper manner.

For them, the trick is going to be with making sure that they are focusing on the most calorie dense foods possible so that they can reach very high intakes without feeling incredibly stuffed and bloated.

If you've ever tried to eat 4000-5000 calories in a day, you know that it can be a real challenge if you aren't choosing your food choices wisely.

In addition to this, these individuals are also going to need to make sure that they are not overdoing the extra activities in their day.

Basically, they want to get into the gym, do a lower volume program that pushes their body to the limits weight-lifting wise, and then get out and allow rest and recovery to take place.

These body types require very little cardio and in fact, doing too much cardio will definitely work against them and their efforts. They must keep cardio training to a minimum.

So the overall guidelines for the ectomorph are essentially opposite that of an endomorph.

- Low volume weight lifting program
- Very little, if any, cardio training
- Ultra-high calorie diet focusing on calorie dense foods of all three macronutrients
- Plenty of rest and recovery time

These individuals should also aim to keep their life as stress free as possible as high levels of stress will also make it harder to recover between their workout sessions and make it even less likely that they see the muscle building results they're after.

Mesomorphs

Finally, we come to the last body type, the mesomorph. Individuals who have this body type are those who tend to have a stockier, muscular build, so they are thick and that is due to muscle mass.

They're often those who were more athletic as kids both because they enjoyed physical activity and because their body type made them naturally excel at sports, thus they enjoyed doing them even more.

These individuals seem to build muscle just by looking at weights and often have a body that is quite resistant to fat gain.

That isn't to say all mesomorphs are resistant to fat gain however, some do tend to pack on body fat if they aren't careful with their food intake they will never pack on body fat as easily as the endomorph does.

These individuals are in the best position because they can include some cardio if they wish and as long as they are doing a relatively intense workout program, this is all they generally need to see muscle growth taking place.

They don't need anything too fancy and tend to respond well to just about any properly structured program.

So for them, it's just a matter of getting the job done.

They need to follow their diet and workout program, making sure sessions don't get skipped and they will be off to seeing results.

Overall, the training and nutrition guidelines for this body type are relatively standard.

- Reasonable calorie intake with a slight deficit for fat loss or a slight surplus for muscle gain
- Mixed diet that's balanced in carbs/fats most of the time (at times, they may go low carb to speed up the rate in which fat is lost)
- Proper strength training workout program
- A few intense cardio sessions per week to keep them lean and enhance their fitness

People in this position should thank their lucky stars because they got a body that they aren't going to have to fight all that hard- not nearly as hard as the endomorphs or ectomorphs.

Taking your own body type into account as you develop your program plan will make sure that you're doing everything properly for <u>you.</u>

So now that you understand the various types of workouts that you can do, let's go on and talk more about why getting fit doesn't need to take hours out of your day.

Chapter 12:
How To Design A Time-Efficient, Effective Workout Program

One of the top excuses that so many people use over and over again as the primary reason why they are unable to reach their fitness goals is simply the lack of time.

You have a million and one things that you need to be doing throughout the day and as much as you may very well want to get that workout in, it just isn't happening.

You figure that if you can't make it to the gym for the full hour session that you have scheduled, there's really no point in going at all and you should instead just accept that you're not cut out for this fitness business stuff.

Not so.

The fact of the matter is that getting fit and leaning down definitely does not need to take hours and hours out of your day – not if you plan your workouts properly and are wise with your diet program.

We've already covered the in's and outs of a good diet protocol, therefore there isn't much more that you need to know about there, but essentially, the greater adherence you have to a proper diet plan, the less overall exercise you'll have to do.

Once again, losing weight is very much about creating that calorie deficit that causes the body to turn to body fat stores as a fuel source and if you're eating well, this is going to be that much easier.

You'll be creating the deficit with the diet therefore you won't need to do a great deal of exercise to try and do it for you.

As we discussed earlier, you will never overcome a bad diet with over exercise, so you really shouldn't even try.

Instead, focus on eating right and exercising wisely to boost your metabolic rate and improve your ability to sustain lean muscle mass.

Those are the two priorities of your workout program and those don't take all that long at all to do. If you can commit just 90 minutes per week to exercising, that's all you really need at minimum.

So all of this said, let's go into what you need to know about designing a workout that is shorter on time, but yet high on results.

Full Body Approach

The very first thing I would recommend you do as you go about setting up a workout program to see optimal results with your fitness goals is utilizing the full body approach.

Why full body?

If you've read many fitness magazines before, you may have come to notice that many people appear to be using a split body approach. They go to the gym and work their chest one day, their shoulders the next day, their arms and triceps following, finishing up with a back day and a legs day.

Isn't that a better option since then you can work each muscle group itself with sole attention during the single session?

Definitely not.

The problem with the split body approach is the fact that it's going to have you working the muscles at a very low frequency level (just once per week) and you won't be stimulating that many muscle fibers in each session you do.

I mean think about it – a biceps and triceps day?

How many muscle fibers could you possibly hit on such a day?

Very, very few – at least in comparison to say a day where you work the legs, shoulders, chest, and back altogether in one session.

 Get an Edge!
With a full body approach, you really only need to be performing 4-5 exercises total if you're really short on time, so this is the absolute best workout for someone who leads a busy lifestyle.

THAT is a total and complete workout that will stimulate so much muscle mass, your metabolism will be supercharged for hours after the workout is completed.

And that is what brings good results.

There are a number of other important benefits to a full body approach as well.

For instance, a full body approach requires a minimal amount of time, yet you still will get to work the muscles at that high frequency level.

You'll hit them three days per week using an on/off/on/off/on/off/off set-up. This not only means greater stimulation, but greater rest as well.

Remember, recovery is vital for success as well. If you aren't recovering between your workout sessions, you won't be seeing progress in any regard because you will just be continually breaking down your muscle tissues further and further.

In addition to that, the full body workout, because it works such large muscle groups in the session, will get your heart rate up so it actually also becomes slightly cardiovascular in nature.

This means you now won't have to do as much cardio training either.

See, it's a win-win approach. So rather than splitting your body up as you go along, hit the entire body hard, then go home and rest. Then go back and repeat all over again.

That will yield the most optimal results for 99% of the population.

Even advanced trainees can see tremendous strength gains with the full body approach so you won't even necessarily have to change the workout structure around as you progress through. As long as you focus on making sure that you are continually adding more weight, changing around the exercises, altering the sets and reps performed and so on, that's all that you'll need to be doing for best results.

Another great thing about the full body approach is that if you do happen to have an extra busy week and can't make it to the gym for one of your sessions, this isn't a big deal because you'll still hit each muscle group twice per week, which is the minimum frequency recommended to keep progress moving along.

With any other workout split and especially the body part split, if you miss a day, you're pretty much not going to hit that particular muscle group all week – which is clearly not an ideal scenario by any means.

So for the workouts in this program, we will be using this method.

Note that the upper/lower approach, where you divide the body up in half and work the upper body on one day, the lower on the next, rest, then repeat before taking the weekend off, can also be a route you could go if you really wanted as you'll still hit each muscle group twice per week and allow for three days of rest overall during the course of the week.

The advantages to that set-up is that you can perform slightly more exercises per muscle group since you only have to get through half the body in the single session, but the disadvantages are that you are in the gym four days per week and you still only hit them twice, not three times like the full body approach.

So you can decide for yourself which you prefer.

Full body is best, upper/lower is still permissible, body part split should be avoided.

Follow this protocol and you'll be setting yourself up for results.

Exercise Selection

The next element that has to get put into place as you design your workout program is the exercise selection that you'll be using.

The exercises that you choose to make your workout up out of can have a significant influence on the results that you see because these will establish what sort of metabolic rate increase you achieve, how much total weight you can lift and therefore the strength gains that you receive, as well as how high your heart rate gets.

Finally, it'll also determine the length of your workout session, which is why we're having this discussion in the first place.

Choose the right exercises and you can easily get in and out of the gym in 20-30 minutes and get in a complete workout session.

Choose the wrong exercises and you'll easily be in there for an hour and you won't even see as good of results as in the former scenario.

So what makes for a good exercise session?

What do you have to do to ensure that you are moving along properly and maximizing every second in the gym? When looking at your exercise selection, you want to be choosing exercises that are going to work as many different muscle groups as possible in a single instant.

Remember, the more muscle groups you can hit in a single movement, the faster your metabolic rate will be and the faster you will see strength gains occurring.

Exercises that achieve this are labeled compound exercises and typically span across two different joints as you perform them.

Examples include:

- Bench Press
- Shoulder Press
- Bent over rows
- Lat pull-downs
- Pull-ups
- Push-ups
- Squats
- Deadlifts
- Lunges
- Step-ups
- Leg press
- Split squats
- Plank exercise

Each of these exercises stimulates at least two muscle groups so you'll be able to hit the entire body faster in each workout session. If you can work all muscles in four exercises versus doing them in 10, which workout gets you in and out quickly?

Hopefully you can see and understand how this works.

Now, this isn't to say that there isn't a place for more isolated exercise. At times, it can be helpful to perform exercises that are going to work just a single muscle group at once.

For instance, if you really want to see increased strength gains and one particular muscle group seems to be lagging and not improving at all, then it can be beneficial to work that muscle group with not only a compound movement, but also an isolation one as well.

This enhanced focus is going to help to improve the total fatigue-factor that muscle experiences during each of your workouts and that higher level of fatigue is what will then help to bring on optimal results.

Isolation exercises can also be good for defining a muscle as you go about a fat loss process and begin getting leaner. If you work the muscle just on its own, you may see slightly more definition and muscular striations occurring then if you just worked it in a compound movement.

Finally, isolation exercises can also be used to help take fatigue up a notch before or after doing a compound movement. This is an advanced technique that can be utilized and one that we will talk about into greater detail shortly when we get to chapter 14.

 Get an Edge!

If you aren't quite sure how to perform any of the resistance training exercises that we're talking about, make sure that you book a session with a personal trainer who can show you. It's imperative that you use good form as you go about your workouts, so do not skip over this no matter what – your success depends on it.

So which are the isolation exercises?

The primary isolation exercises that you'll come into include:

- Bicep curls
- Tricep extensions
- Lateral raises
- Front raises

- Rear delt raises
- Leg extensions
- Hamstring curls
- Calf raises

See how these all work just that single muscle group? That's what makes them an isolation exercise.

These should typically always be added towards the end of a workout session unless you are using them through one of the advanced techniques that we'll be discussing shortly.

Finally, the last thing that you must keep in mind and remember at all times with regards to exercise selection is that it has to be well-balanced and at an appropriate volume level.

You cannot go off doing ten different compound exercises in a single workout and expect to feel your best over the course of time.

That will be a quick route to overtraining, which believe me, you do not want to get yourself into. We'll talk more about that in a coming chapter as well.

Balance is key and as you go about working out and learning how your body is responding to various workout protocols, you will come to see how much you can tolerate.

Some individuals will easily be able to do 30 sets per workout session while others may only be able to do 20 before fatigue hits and they have to get out and start the recovery process.

By paying attention to the signs and signals that your body is demonstrating, you can ensure that you are going to be optimizing your progress and moving forward as you had hoped.

Reps/Sets

Moving along, the next element that will need to be considered as you design your workout protocol is the reps and sets that you are performing. These have a direct influence over how much total volume you're doing in each workout session, so again have to be lined up properly if you are going to be seeing optimal results and preventing overtraining.

In addition to that, they are also going to have an immediate influence over how much weight you can lift as you move through the workout and that again is going to be a determining factor of the type of progress that you see.

First let's talk about reps.

How many reps you perform is correlated with how much weight you're lifting as just mentioned. The more reps you have to perform, obviously the less weight you'll be able to lift overall.

Likewise, the fewer reps you perform, the more weight you should be able to lift since you can go full out and hit that point of fatigue sooner.

So depending on your own goals and preferences, you can adjust the rep range as required.

If you want to see maximum strength gains, the typical rep range to use is in the neighborhood of 3-6 reps. 3 is very low and will only be for more advanced individuals, so typically aim for 5-6 reps.

If you're someone who wants to build both strength and more muscle size, then you need to be in the 'hypertrophy' rep range, which is going to have you lifting at 6-10 reps. 8-10 is most ideal here for most individuals.

Beyond 10 reps you'll move into the muscular endurance goal set and this range can be beneficial, but note there are limits. I would never recommend taking your reps much higher than 15, unless you are doing a specific protocol such as timed reps or you are actually just trying to do a set until complete and total fatigue.

Otherwise, beyond 15 reps, you're going to have to lighten the weight so much that it's not really going to be all that beneficial for you any more at all, therefore it can hinder the progress that you see.

Remember that the whole point of strength training is to lift enough weight and if you're lightening the load so much because you are aiming for 20-30 reps, you aren't building much strength.

All you'll really get out of such a workout is a bit of fatigue occurring.

Also keep in mind that the compound exercises are typically the ones that you will perform using the lower rep range as they are the primary strength builders while the isolation exercises will typically have you moving into the higher rep range instead.

Very rarely will you ever find a workout protocol calling for five reps of a bicep curl for instance, however it's not abnormal at all to see a protocol listing five reps of a chest press.

The chest press is a primary strength building exercise because you're again going to work so many muscle fibers while you do it, therefore you will want to lift maximally and this by nature means you will decrease the total reps performed.

So that now covers the reps that you're doing, what about sets?

The total number of sets you're doing is also something that does need to be taken into account if you wish to move forward and succeed with your program.

When factoring in sets, you'll want to be thinking about the exercise you're doing, the total number of reps you're performing, as well as how many exercises you're doing in the workout overall.

If you are doing five exercises total and perform five sets of each exercise, that translates to 25 sets overall – which is a fairly good range for most people.

If on the other hand you're doing ten exercises and attempt to do five sets in all of those exercises as well, now you're at 50 sets overall, which is going to be way too much for almost all individuals to manage.

Most people will do best in the range of 20 sets per workout for those who have a very poor recovery system and often find themselves fatiguing quickly up to 35 sets per workout for those who recover very well and can take a higher amount of volume (usually it's younger males who have plenty of testosterone flowing through their body that will be able to go up to this level).

Everyone else will want to aim for around 25-30 sets per workout.

Get an Edge!

If you decrease the total amount of rest you take between your sets, you can forgo cardio training entirely because you will be getting a cardiovascular workout with the strength training session that you're doing.

One factor that also influences this set range however is the total reps that you're doing as well. If you're performing five reps for instance, you will be doing more sets overall than if you're doing 12 reps per set.

The general rule of thumb to follow here is that you want to land somewhere in the 24-30 rep range as well.

So if you're doing 5 reps per set, you could do 5 sets total.

If you're doing 8 reps per set, you could do 3 sets total.

If you're doing 12 reps per set, aim for 2.

Again, remember that it's typically compound exercises that you take in the lower rep range and isolation exercises that you'll take higher, so it works out well in that you'll end up doing more total sets per workout of compound moves than isolation moves, which is the way it should be as these exercises are the ones that will form the foundation of your workout protocol.

Of course if you are really pressed for time and don't have 30 minutes to do a workout session, then you will want to be taking your total set range downward.

If you do 1-2 maximum effort sets per exercise, you can still create a very powerful workout that's going to have you still seeing good progress but getting out of the gym in 10-15 minutes.

You should never decrease the total number of exercises in a session if you want to get done faster as you want to make sure that you hit each and every muscle group in all the sessions that you do.

Decreasing the total sets performed with each exercise is the far superior route to take.

Rest Periods

Finally, the last element that you'll want to take into account is the rest periods that you're using as you move through the workout period.

Rest periods are going to be critical for your success as these will dictate how cardiovascular focused the workout is, how much weight you can lift with each set you do (as the more weight you have to lift, the more time you will require for recovery) and of course, how long the workout takes.

The longer your rest periods are, the longer you are going to have to be in the gym, so this is something that you clearly do need to be mindful about.

Rest periods can range significantly from zero seconds all the way up to a maximum of three minutes if you were lifting as heavy of a weight as you possibly could.

Those who want to focus on pure strength and nothing else and plan to work most exercises in the 3-5 rep range (so basically they are maxing out), should be taking rest periods of about 2 ½ to 3 minutes long.

Note that there's no real benefit to resting longer than three minutes so don't ever let it go beyond that. Keep a timer on hand if you have to so that you can monitor your rest periods.

On the other end of the spectrum, circuit training is going to have you forgoing rest periods and moving from one exercise to the next until a series has been completed upon which you will then rest for recovery before possibly completing the circuit once again (depending on the specific workout protocol that you're doing).

Supersets, which are an advanced technique we'll be talking about shortly are another place where rest will be eliminated between two workouts.

For regular workout protocols however, you'll typically want to be around the 30-90 second mark. The heavier the weight and the lower the rep range, the shorter the rest period will be.

Likewise, isolation exercises can typically always have shorter rest periods than compound movements because they're working fewer muscle fibers total so won't get your heart rate up as much and take as long to recover from.

Here's a good rule of thumb to use.

Compound exercises in the slightly higher rep range (8-12 reps): 45-60 seconds rest

Compound exercises in the lower rep range (5-8 reps): 60-90 seconds rest

Isolation exercises in the lower rep range (8-10 reps): 60 seconds rest

Isolation exercises in the higher rep range (10-15 reps): 20-30 seconds rest

Follow these guidelines with a bit of alteration and you will be structuring things properly.

Note thought that shorter rest periods should never cause you to sacrifice proper form. If you are not maintaining proper form during any given exercise, you are making a critical mistake so this must be avoided at all costs.

Form is of utmost importance so focus on that first. If your rest period is up and you still feel slightly fatigued, take a bit more time until you feel ready to go again. You're better off using a bit more rest and then continuing on than you are going forward immediately and pulling a muscle or significantly injuring yourself because you used poor form.

So there you have the main elements of workout program design to be taking into account as you move forward with structuring a workout routine.

While this may feel slightly overwhelming at first and like a lot to take in, rest assured that once you get started designing a protocol, it'll all come together nicely and you shouldn't have any problem piecing together what you need to.

And of course I've made things incredibly easy and have put together a full workout protocol to be following in the third part of this book.

So now that you know how to design a time efficient, effective workout program, let's move forward and talk more about how to set up a home gym properly for those who don't want to workout in the commercial gym setting.

CHAPTER 13:
Setting Up A Home Gym

When it comes to getting your workouts in, you really need to make sure that you weigh your personal preferences so that you can determine which environment is most likely to keep you coming back for more.

The single most important determinant of whether you continue to see progress with your workout program is whether you continue to do it. Period. If you don't do the workouts, you don't get results. It's that simple.

For many people, the commercial gym environment is very intimidating and there are a number of drawbacks involved.

Some of these include:

- Expensive gym membership fees
- Busy environment that means you have to wait for equipment
- Uncomfortable around some of the other members attending the gym
- Long drives to and from the gym
- Limited operating hours

For some people, all of these drawbacks are enough to deter them from getting the workouts in, which is precisely what you don't want.

Enter the home gym.

The home gym offers many advantages since it'll allow you to workout when you want in the privacy of your own home and there will be zero waiting around for equipment.

For those who work irregular hours or find they have a very limited time to get a workout in and thus can't afford to drive 20 minutes to and from the commercial gym, the home gym might be the only solution.

Some people are also under the belief that you can't get an effective workout in at home unless you have a high amount of fancy equipment, but that's not the case at all.

 Get an Edge!
Want to stick to a budget? Be sure to check out second hand gym equipment. You can often find the equipment that you need at a greatly cost-reduced price, so this can make setting up your home gym much more feasible. Just be careful when purchasing cardio equipment that you do give it a test run beforehand to ensure it's working properly.

Let's look at some of the primary equipment options to consider as you design and set up your own home gym.

Cardio Options

First you'll want to get a method in for doing cardio training.

If you're on a really limited budget and live in a location that has stairs, those can make for a fantastic option to get you going. Nothing is going to get your heart rate up and have you burning up calories faster than running up and down a flight of stairs.

Of course, there's also the great outdoors. Depending on where you live and how safe you feel running in your area, you can easily head outside and get your cardio in that way, cycling, walking, or running.

The third indoor option is skipping. A simple skipping rope costs a mere $10 and will provide you with a better workout than running would, so this option should not be overlooked either.

Of course you will need a relatively open space to do the skipping.

If you're more into aerobics, consider one of the cardio workout videos available. Whether it's kickboxing, zumba, or some other variety, there are plenty of options out there for you to choose from.

Last but not least, don't overlook dancing. As silly as it may sound, if you crank up your favorite music and start to dance with full effort, this can be an incredibly great full body workout that sends your calorie burn soaring.

So there you have some of the key very low cost ways to get in your cardio workout.

Of course if you do have a higher budget, then you may want to look into the cardio machine equipment options available. Treadmills, bikes, ellipticals, and so on.

These are going to run you more budget-wise, but if you make a good investment they can last you for years.

Strength Training Options

Once you have your cardio option set, it's time to look at the strength training options.

At the very low cost level (basically free!) you have the bodyweight exercises. Now, you can do these and get in an effective workout when you're just starting, but note that as you progress along, you may find that you need to start adding more external resistance in order to keep the progress coming along.

So while bodyweight exercises can be effective for the beginner, they likely won't be fully effective for the more advanced individual.

At that point, you'll need more.

Now, resistance bands can make for a good option and are quite cost-effective as well. They'll be around $20-50 in most places depending on the variety you purchase and this will provide that external resistance. T

They also tuck away into a drawer when not in use, so are a good option for those who are more limited in terms of how much space they have.

On the drawback side of things, they won't provide as much resistance as weights will, so eventually they may no longer be challenging either.

But as a progression model, they can definitely get the job done.

Finally, you then have free weights – dumbbells and plate weight. These are going to be the ideal option and what I would highly recommend that you do pick up.

An exchangeable set of dumbbells will help ensure that you aren't taking up much space in your home and allow you to customize your workout based on how much weight you need.

If you are getting more advanced and have the room available, you can also look into a barbell along with a bench press and squat machine with plate weight.

This is going to be a very effective manner to train as with these three pieces of equipment (bench, squat rack, and dumbbells), you can easily do absolutely everything you could possibly need for an effective workout.

If you get these, you will never need to purchase anything else equipment-wise unless you want to.

Finally, for those who prefer not using free weights and using weight machines instead, you can get one of those universal gym systems that comes with chest presses, shoulder presses, lat pull-downs, leg extensions, and so on.

These can be a good option as well if you do prefer that. Many people do tend to be limited by room with this option and budget can become a concern (some are quite pricey), but that option is there if you really want to step things up and build a complete home gym.

So there you have the main requirements of building an effective home gym. As you can see, you can really build a gym on any budget level and create an effective workout with it.

The key is just thinking about your experience level and what you want out of your workout session.

So now that we've talked about this, let's move forward and go over some advanced theories of training to know about as you continue to progress along.

CHAPTER 14:
Progression Techniques To Take Your Workout Up A Notch

For the very beginners, simply focusing on straight sets as you build the foundation of strength in your body is going to be the route to go. There's no need to do anything too fancy early on – you simply need to focus on lifting more and more weight over time.

But after you've been at it for five to six months, you may be itching to get a bit more advanced and add more excited to your workout program – not to mention a challenge.

That's where some advanced moves can come into play.

By using them, you can kick your workout up a notch and ensure that optimal progression takes place.

Lets' go through what some of these advanced moves are.

Supersets

The first advanced technique is the superset. With this technique, rather than performing one exercise, resting, performing your next set, resting some more and so on, you are going to perform two exercises immediately back to back with each other.

So you'll do one, the next, and then rest before starting the process again.

You can pair together any two exercises you prefer using this technique, however it's typically best to choose either an upper and lower exercise or two that work opposing muscle groups (such as the biceps and triceps for instance).

This way you can get a strong muscle pump going and while one muscle group is working, the other is resting.

Supersets are also going to keep your heart rate up higher as well, so can provide a good metabolic enhancement.

Drop Sets

The next advanced technique is the drop set. Drop sets are also going to be great for helping to ensure that you are pushing through any strength plateaus as it will force your body to work harder than it's used to.

To perform these, you will complete your typical set an then once that set is completed, drop the weight by five to ten pounds. Then complete a second set, and then drop the weight once more until you are at a point of complete exhaustion.

This is a good technique to use when you just can't seem to lift more weight on your usual exercise because after so long of doing this, when you do go back to the straight sets again, you should find that you can kick things up a notch and lift more as your body is used to overcoming fatigue and has gotten stronger.

Just do keep in mind that drop sets are very intense so you won't want to do too many of them per workout session. If you do, you are going to be quite likely to start overtraining or suffer from poor recovery.

 Get an Edge!
Drop sets are a perfect way to boost muscle definition before any special event you have coming up, so if you want instant leanness and to look more toned, this is the method to add to your workouts.

Sets For Time

Sets for time is the next advanced technique to consider. With sets for time, you're going to perform as many reps as you can in a certain time frame – typically about a minute. The advantage to doing this is that you will push past fatigue and train your body for muscular endurance.

I don't recommend you do this all the time, but at various points in the program it can help you kick your results up a notch and help to give your body something new to deal with.

For these sets, you don't want to go too light on the weight however. Keep the weight at the standard level that challenges you at about 10-12 reps and then simply take very brief rest periods as needed throughout that minute.

It's a must you maintain proper form throughout so if you feel fatigue, pause for a very brief second and then carry on once again.

Once the minute is up, then you can go forward and take the rest you need.

Sets for time is also a great way to get your heart rate up, so yet another one of those techniques to consider to get cardio training in as well.

Pre-Fatigue Sets

Finally, the last of the advanced techniques that you will want to consider are pre-fatigue sets. These are going to be sets where you tire out one muscle through an isolation exercise before performing a primary compound movement.

So let's say you want to focus on the chest muscle.

Since the triceps are assistors to the chest when doing a bench press and will, by nature, take some stress off the chest when you perform that movement, you want to tire them out so they no longer are helping.

So you'd perform a few sets of a tricep isolation exercise such as tricep extensions for instance and then go on and perform your bench press.

In doing so you will then fully work the chest muscle and over time, it'll get stronger. Then when you go back to doing the straight chest workout, no tricep isolation exercise done first, you should be able to lift more weight.

Just like the other advanced protocols, these are very intense as well, so aim to just do one or two per workout session.

And note that with all of these advanced techniques, you typically will not use more than one at a time either, but instead you'll want to alternate between them as you go.

So there you have the advanced exercises that will help you take things up to the next level. They will all add more interest and excitement to your program, while helping you see maximum fitness.

Now let's talk about what would happen however if you do too many of these advanced exercises or are not smart in your approach and move on to suffer from a state of overtraining.

CHAPTER 15:
Overtraining 101

One of the most problematic issues that could occur as you go about your workout program is dealing with overtraining. Far too many individuals come to think that overtraining will only happen to serious athletes who are training as a career, but that is not the case at all.

In fact, overtraining is almost more likely to happen to new exercisers because your body has not yet adapted to the stress of training yet an because you may not be using all the nutritional an recovery techniques you could be.

So let's walk you through some information on what overtraining is and how you can best manage an prevent it – and what to do if you begin to suffer.

What Is Overtraining?

First things first, let's get into what overtraining is so that you can fully understand how this happens and how it will impact you.

Overtraining is essentially a state where you're placing more demands on the body than what it's able to cope with. Each and every day, your body has so many resources at its disposal to deal with the stressors that it's going to be facing.

If you lead a very high-paced and stressful life, you'll be depleting these resources naturally each day. Then, you go to bed at night and you recover, restoring your resource level.

But, when you start adding intense training to the mix, now you have a whole other element that's putting a very high level of stress on the body.

How much stress is being place depends primarily on the intensity of the exercise. If you go out for a 20 minute walk at lunch, this really won't be all that stressful at all and you'll likely recover without a hitch. It won't impact you and you'll continue feeling fine.

But, if you hit the gym and do 20 minutes of intense weight lifting in circuit training fashion, you can rest assured you've just placed a great deal more stress on the body and have used up some of those limited resources that your body has to deal with this stress.

If you're doing too much and reaching a state of depletion – possibly trying to do more when in that depleted state, that's when overtraining occurs.

Basically, it would be like emptying the gas tank in a car and then trying to keep driving. You aren't going to get very far and that car is likely to break down.

The same goes for your body.

As soon as you drain your recovery reserves, the minute you continually ask your body to keep performing at an optimal level, it's going to falter and you're going to wind up not feeling so well.

Do this for a long enough period of time and that's when overtraining is going to set in.

Get an Edge!

One of the best things that you can do to prevent over-training is to keep your day to day stress levels lower so that you aren't releasing cortisol throughout the body due to stress. Practice deep breathing, take a long bath, or book a massage. Do whatever it takes to get your stress levels under control.

So to summarize, overtraining is a state of miss-match. It's a state of dishing out more stress on an ongoing basis than your body is designed to handle.

Overtraining isn't going to take place in just one day. One day of overdoing things will leave you tired and a little less energetic the next day, but it's not going to push you into a state of full blown overtraining.

Do this for seven days in a row though and you're going to be walking a fine line.

Do it for two weeks in a row and you won't be doing your next workouts. The body needs rest and recovery and if you're not willingly giving it, it will get it from you another way (by causing overtraining to set in).

That's the basics of overtraining. Now, overtraining can be divided into two different types however and understanding the differences in them is important.

CNS Overtraining

The very first type of overtraining is CNS overtraining. CNS stands for central nervous system so this is a case of placing too much overall strain on your body. With CNS overtraining, it doesn't especially matter what type of activity you're doing, it's just a matter of you doing too much activity that is too intense in nature.

To put this into perspective, imagine this scenario.

You've designed a workout program for yourself that's going to span over a five day period.

It looks like this:

Monday – you'll train chest

Tuesday - you'll train back

Wednesday – you'll train legs

Thursday – you'll train shoulders

Friday – you'll train arms

Weekend – you'll finally rest

Now, at first glance, you may think that this set-up is fine. After all, each muscle group has more than 48 hours to rest, which is the often stated requirement in order to prevent over training.

So you begin the program thinking that you're on the way to fast results.

Only, by the time Wednesday hits, your leg workout is suffering. You're actually weaker on the main lifts that you're planning on doing compared to what you were last week.

What gives?

Your legs should be fully rested so they should be stronger not less powerful.

The problem here is that your CNS is tired. You've done two intense workouts before it – chest and back and that has placed great strain on your system.

What you must remember is that your CNS is responsible for strength output. It doesn't matter if you're doing a bicep curl or a bent over row, you will be stressing out the CNS whenever you ask it to lift a heavy load.

So despite the fact that your muscles will be well rested, your CNS, which is what generates the force needed to move a weight is not. Therefore, your workouts begin to suffer.

This is why complete rest days are so critical. It doesn't matter if you're doing different types of workouts working different muscle groups throughout the week, if you aren't giving your body a chance to recharge CNS-wise, you aren't going to be making progress.

So the main point to note here is that it's not enough to just be making sure each muscle group has 48 hours to rest. You also need to make sure that your CNS has time off throughout the week as well.

Muscular Overtraining

Now the next type of overtraining that you need to also be paying attention to is muscular overtraining. This is the type of overtraining that is prevented by following the rule, 'Never work the same muscle group within 48 hours'.

So basically, you can't go into the gym and perform leg weight training exercises on Monday and do the exact same thing on Tuesday.

If you do that, you're going to be hindering your ability to recover and will likely only break down the muscle tissues further rather than building them up stronger as you had hoped you would.

Muscular overtraining is the type of overtraining that most people think of when they hear the word 'overtraining' but is actually the least common of the two.

Most of those participating in any sort of workouts will have done some background reading on overtraining and will realize the importance of the 48 hour rule.

It's far more common for individuals to be over-excited about their workout and going to the gym daily or starting to feel guilty if they don't do some form of intense exercise each and every day.

For that reason, it's CNS overtraining that is the more likely issue.

Nevertheless, care must be paid to making absolute certain that you are giving your muscles enough rest between sessions.

One fact that some people will tend to overlook is that certain exercises are going to work more than one muscle group at once, so you have to be very careful with your workout programming.

For example, if you did a chest workout one day and thought you could do a arms workout the next and then take your day off to prevent CNS overtraining, you're still at risk for muscular overtraining.

Since when you do your chest workout you're essentially going to be working the chest, shoulders, as well as the tricep sand biceps, the arms workout the next day will not be giving these muscles the 48 hours of rest that they need.

Thus, they won't be recovered and you'll end up breaking them down rather than building them up.

This is how muscular overtraining very often starts out. Poor workout planning is the biggest reason it will occur.

Fortunately, muscular overtraining does tend to be the easier form of overtraining to recover from because it's not systemic in nature. CNs is going to impact your entire body, whereas muscular overtraining is only going to impact one specific area.

This is why with CNS overtraining, it doesn't matter which muscle groups you're working, you're still going to feel tired.

With muscular overtraining, you could very likely train other muscle groups and feel fine, but when you're training the one that's been impacted, you're going to notice that you're not nearly as strong as you were before.

Who Is Most Likely To Overtrain?

So now that we've introduced the two main types of overtraining, it's time to address who is most likely to overtrain in the first place. This is another important thing to consider because it's going to influence whether or not you need to be paying more attention to this in the first place.

So who are the people who are most at risk?

While each and every individual will have their own training capacity tolerance, so it will vary from person to person, there are some general guidelines to follow.

Here's what to note.

Older Individuals

Older individuals (40 years and older) tend to have lower rates of recovery abilities as their body doesn't 'bounce back' as quickly, so will be more likely to overtrain.

When you're younger, your body is fairly resilient to training stresses and your immune system will be working at top level function.

As you get older however, your immune system isn't as strong and your body simply can't handle as much as it used to.

For this reason, workout frequency will need to be cut back. You want to avoid cutting back on the intensity however as this is what makes a workout effective in the first place.

Those Leading Stressful Lifestyles

Those who lead very stressful lifestyles will already be taxing their body to an extreme extent, so with the addition of intense workouts, this is more likely to put them over the edge.

If you're hardly recovering from your day to day tasks as it is, if you start to add additional exercise into the mix, this could be what it takes to move you to a state of overtraining.

This can occur the other way around as well. If you're doing your workout program and are feeling fine – fatigued on some days but generally good overall, but then something very stressful happens in your life, say you are struggling financial or are going through relationship problems, the extra stress added will not move you to a state of overtraining.

Earlier your workouts were fine with your low-stress lifestyle but now, they're just too much. This is why constantly monitoring your day to day lifestyle along with your workouts is important.

If you're going to through a very busy and stressful period in your life, it might be worthwhile to consider cutting back on your workouts slightly so that they don't get to be a problem for the time being.

Dieting Individuals

The next person who will be at a much higher risk for overtraining is those who are currently on a fat loss diet. Any time you reduce your calorie intake below where it's supposed to be, you're not going to be providing your body as much fuel as it would ideally like.

Since it takes energy to complete the recovery and repair process, if you aren't giving your body this energy, you can't expect it to recover nearly as well.

One of the first very important rules when you go on a diet is to start cutting back on your workout intensity. Fail to do this and you're headed for trouble.

This is also why your protein needs will go up when dieting, as we'll look at more thoroughly in the nutrition section of the book. When you're using a fat loss diet plan and performing intense workouts, there is a greater chance that protein may be utilized as a fuel source, leaving less protein left over to sustain proper muscle repair and maintenance.

If your muscles aren't getting the protein that they need, this only means one thing: lean muscle mass loss.

To avoid that, protein needs go up so that if some is burned off as a fuel source, you'll still be able to sustain enough to keep your muscles intact.

When dieting it's going to be especially important that you're also paying attention to all the other recovery strategies that you should be doing as well as each of these will help you in your fight against overtraining.

 Get an Edge!

If you are going to go on a very strict diet, be sure to cut back on your exercise volume to ensure that you are able to recover between each workout session that you do.

Females

While it's not always the case, in general, most women will have slightly lower recovery capacities compared to males. Females have less testosterone, which is the primary hormone that is involved in physical activity and muscle building.

This is completely normal and natural and there isn't really anything that you can do about this fact beyond accepting it and adjusting your training protocol to accommodate.

Females should be more careful about making sure to have sufficient easy days in their workout program along with at least one full rest day per week.

Interestingly to note, when women go on a fat loss diet and overdo it with the exercise, their bodies are also far more likely to fight them, causing the metabolic rate to slow down and actually holding onto body fat stores.

This is in part due to the fact that females have a higher necessary body fat requirement in order to give birth so any time you threaten to decrease body fat, the body gets alarmed much more quickly.

Males can push the barrier a little further before problems start setting in. Females will run into problems.

So there you have the primary people who will be at risk for overtraining. If you are in a high risk group, this doesn't necessarily mean that it's definitely going to happen to you.

As long as you learn proper preventative methods, you can definitely avoid this from taking place and continue on with your workout program without any issues whatsoever.

Now let's move forward and speak a little more about the symptoms of overtraining that you need to be on the lookout for.

Symptoms Of Overtraining

Perhaps one of the absolute best preventative strategies that you need to take note of as far as avoiding overtraining is learning the signs and symptoms that will occur that indicate that you're moving to a place of being overtrained.

Often the symptoms won't come on suddenly, but rather they'll continue to build over time until they finally get so great that you just cannot continue on with your workouts any longer.

Also important to note is that you may not experience all the symptoms either. Some people will experience overtraining differently than others, so it's not a one-size-fits-all phenomenon.

Two people may have completely different symptoms, but if left ignored, will end up in the exact same place – overtrained and unable to continue on with their workouts.

So what are the main symptoms that you need to be on the lookout for?

The symptoms can be broken down into training related symptoms that you experience while you're training and then symptoms that impact your everyday life and that you struggle to deal with on an ongoing basis.

Let's have a look at the ones to note.

Physical Symptoms:

- Slower recovery than normal after workouts are performed
- Frequent and ongoing muscle soreness that never legs up
- The development of nagging injuries that keep you from your workouts
- Lower workout performance – either reduced strength capacity or lower levels of endurance
- Higher resting heart rate, especially upon waking
- Greater frequency of illnesses of infections, indicating a reduce immune system capacity
- Difficulty sleeping – either falling asleep or staying asleep
- Increased irritability and anxiety
- Feeling tired all the time like you want to sleep all day long
- Weight changes, either gained or lost without intension
- Appetite changes, either increasing or decreasing
- Decreased insulin sensitivity
- Decreased testosterone production
- Increased cortisol production

Psychological Symptoms

In addition to the physical symptoms presented above, the following psychological symptoms may manifest themselves as well.

- Depression or strong feelings of being sad and down
- Lost of interest in activities formerly enjoyed
- Very little joy in daily activities; loss of vigor
- Low libido levels
- Very low desire to perform any sort of training

As you can see, overtraining really can impact all areas of your life, so it's important not to take this lightly.

Again, remember that these symptoms may come on to be rather minor at first. You may initially note that you're feeling a little down and 'on edge'. In addition to that, your workouts may not be going as planned, which you chalk up to the reason of why you are agitated.

But, as time progresses and your workouts continually take a turn for the worse, you may start seeing other symptoms come on as well. At this point, you know you're on a bad path and effort must be made immediately to remedy the situation.

Don't wait until the symptoms are in their full glory to do something about this. Take action immediately when you first notice them occurring. If you do that, you're going to stand a far better chance of preventing overtraining before it starts.

So now that you know the symptoms to watch out for, let's go over some of the methods that you can use to prevent over-training in the first place.

Preventing Overtraining

In addition to watching out for the primary symptoms of over-training and doing something about it the minute you notice them occurring, there are some additional things that you can do further to help reduce the chances that this problem impacts you.

Remember, prevention will always be the best medicine. If you avoid letting overtraining develop, you'll side step potentially having to take weeks if not months off to get yourself back up to speed.

Let's have a look at the main methods that you must keep in mind at all times.

Workout Structure

The very first thing that you'll need to take a good look at is the workout structure that you're using. Are you giving yourself enough total days off each week to rest?

Are you including some easier days in your training week along with your more intense days?

Are you making sure that you give each muscle group the 48 hours of rest it needs between sessions, including for the compound exercise-multi-muscle issue? (working more than one muscle group on compound exercises)

If you aren't, it's time to make some changes in your workout schedule.

If you are unsure how to make these changes yourself, it's a good idea to consult with a personal trainer to help you.

Keep in mind as well that even if a workout is not extremely intense in nature, it can still add up and along with the intense workouts you are doing, could become too much.

If you are suffering from a situation where you think that your other activities – perhaps some recreational sports games you play throughout the week are leading you to become over trained with your more intense sessions, then your best interests will be, as long as you are okay with it, cutting those out first.

 Get an Edge!
To check your workout volume, you'll want to multiply the total number of weight you're lifting in each set by the number of reps completed. Do this for each set in the workout and then add them all up to get your grand total – this is the amount of volume you're using.

Everyday Stress

The second preventative measure that you can take to help reduce the chances that you end up becoming overtrained is to look at your everyday stress level.

How stressful is your life on a day to day basis?

Remember that everything will cause stress to build up.

Relationship stress counts.

Financial stress counts.

Career stress counts.

Even simply having a busy schedule on a day to day basis with no change of let-up can prove to be enough stress to push you over the edge.

If you're leading a very stressful life, one of the best preventative methods you can use is to either look at more constructive coping methods to dealing with this stress or look at how you can eliminate some of the things in your life that are causing you all of this stress.

Most people don't have very good stress management techniques and just continue to let stress build up higher and higher until they're at a point where it's impacting them so much they're totally burnt out.

While your intense workout sessions can be great for stress reducing properties themselves, it's important to have some other coping techniques in your arsenal as well.

This could include things such as:

- Scheduling regular days (or even a few hours) for yourself to do something you enjoy
- Utilizing hot baths, which can also help improve recovery
- Scheduling coffee with a good friend to talk about whatever is stressing you
- Using a stress journal so you can get your thoughts out
- Talking to a counselor if there are particular issues you're stressing about that are serious enough to warrant this
- Taking part in relaxation focused exercise sessions such as Hatha yoga
- Making your life as uncluttered as possible
- Learning to say 'no' so that you don't have an overbooked schedule, spreading yourself too thin

All of these can help you get your stress level under control so that it's no longer impacting you and putting you at risk of overtraining.

Proper Nutrition

The next key element to preventing overtraining is taking a good look at your nutrition as well. We will be devoting much more discussion to the proper principles of good nutrition that you need to be following in the next section of the book, but right now let's talk about a few that are of particular importance with regards to preventing overtraining.

The very first thing that you need to be very aware of is your carbohydrate intake. By far, this is one thing that can have the biggest influence on whether or not you move into a state of overtraning.

Attempt too many intense sessions while following a low carb diet plan and you can be assured that you will quickly become overtrained.

In order to perform strength training or interval exercise, glucose must be present in your system. Simply put, without glucose, the muscles will not have the fuel substrate available to perform those workouts.

So if you're using a low calorie, low carb diet, not only are you not providing enough fuel to get through the workout sessions, but you aren't providing enough carbs either.

Fatigue will set in very shortly and shortly thereafter, you simply won't have enough 'juice' in you to complete the workout sessions.

Performance will falter and you'll be on a fast track to few results.

So number one is making sure that you are eating enough carbohydrates before and after your sessions. You can use lower carb dieting the rest of the time but around the workout, carbs need to be there.

Second you have your overall calorie intake. While it may be tempting to adopt a very low calorie diet plan and try and lose weight as quickly as possibly if weight loss is your goal, if you're also interested in doing some intense sessions, you should be avoiding this.

Too low of a calorie intake with so many intense workouts is really going to backfire on you and work against you. You'd think that it'll help you move forward faster, but really, it's going to do the opposite.

You need to be very careful with your diet protocol and be sure that you're fueling yourself enough to get through the workouts.

You will still have to be using a reduced calorie intake with your training in order to see fat loss taking place, but at the same rate, you can't go too low if you expect to sustain your workout program.

Of particular importance with regards to your nutrition is making sure that you're following a very good post workout protocol. We talked about how important carbs are, at this point, the sooner after your workout you can take in both carbs and protein, the better.

It's these two nutrients acting together that will give you the best chance of making a full recovery.

Additionally, cycling your calories over time, that is using higher calorie periods with lower calorie periods is often the best way to do things as this will ensure that you aren't going too long for too long and will also serve to keep your metabolic rate moving along more quickly as well.

Remember that dieting itself is a stress for the body and as we discussed earlier, all stress needs to be reduced and managed.

Good Recovery Habits

Finally, the last thing that you can do to help prevent over-training from taking place is to make sure that you are using as many recovery enhancing techniques available to you. There are a number of things that you can do apart from good nutrition to ensure that you are making the most of your down time between workouts.

Let's go over some of these.

Hot Baths

The very first thing that you should be doing is looking at taking hot baths on a regular basis. The benefit to hot baths are that they will help to increase the rate of blood circulation taking place through the body and the enhanced circulation is going to increase the delivery of oxygen and nutrients to the muscle cells.

Since the muscles are most in need of nutrients post-workout to help rebuild their broken down muscle tissues, this can go a long way towards improving your recovery abilities.

In general, hot baths are also great for stress relieving purposes, as we mentioned above when talking about stress, so that's yet another reason to utilize them.

Foam Rolling

Foam rolling is a newer recovery strategy that more and more people are getting into that will help to reduce muscle soreness and improve your recovery rate.

If you ever find that you're incredibly tense and tight after a workout session, foam rolling may just do the trick to help you out.

The nice thing about foam rolling is that it allows you to specifically pinpoint certain regions in the body and put extra pressure on them, working through their built up stress and causing the muscle fibers to contract and then relax.

Foam rolling will take some practice to learn how to do it correctly, but after some time is spent learning the concept, it's an incredibly effective way to increase your workout recovery.

Elite athletes often use this protocol so if they're using it, it will work great for your HIIT sessions as well.

 Get This!

Each person is going to respond slightly differently to the various recovery strategies so be sure that you are taking this into account as you choose which to use for yourself. Try a few and see which helps you feel the best as you go about your workout session.

Sleep

Moving along, sleep is the next must that you need to be considering for your recovery strategies. Getting a full eight hours of sleep each night will be imperative to allowing you to make a good recovery and is going to help you to feel well rested and ready to attack the next day's session as well.

During the sleep hours your body will go into deep recovery mode and this s also when growth hormone will be released in its highest concentration during the day. Growth hormone is a hormone that is largely responsible for ensuring that you are able to build muscle up as you should and for just increasing the overall recovery process as best as possible as well.

One thing that you should note is that due to your natural circadian rhythm, the hours of sleep that you get before midnight are going to be the hours that are most effective for repair and recovery purposes, so if you can, aim to get to bed sooner rather than later.

You'll see better overall recovery sleeping on a schedule of 10 pm – 6 am than you would on a sleep schedule of 2 am to 10 am. Some people won't have the luxury of going to bed and waking so late in the first place, but if you are someone who does, error on the side of earlier rather than later. You'll get better results from it.

Massage

Going for periodic massages is yet another way to increase the recovery rates that you experience between your workout sessions. Again, these are a bit more of a luxury strategy as there will be a fee involved, but if you are able to spend the money, it will be well worth it.

Massage can be a great way to loosen up tense muscle fibers, improving flexibility, decreasing soreness, improving blood circulation, and will also have a number of positive benefits on your stress level as well.

All in all, it's great all around regardless of the type of physical training you're doing, but for those involved with intense training, it tends to be especially beneficial.

Stretching

Finally, the last recovery strategy that you should be making use of is stretching. Stretching is going to be important to be doing after each workout session you perform as this will help to decrease your risk of developing post-workout muscle soreness and for also helping to bring the heart rate back down to a lower level again, preventing blood pooling in the extremities.

In addition to the five to ten minutes of stretching you do post-workout, it would also be beneficial to be performing some more thorough stretching sessions throughout the week as well.

These will not only help to speed up recovery, but also increase your flexibility as well, which can then assist with reducing the chances that you become sore and tight in the first place.

The more flexible you are, the more you'll be able to handle moving throughout the various range of motions that different exercises call for and the better you'll be able to deal with training demands.

Stretching sessions should always begin with a five minute light warm-up to ensure the muscles are warm and you should be aiming to hold each stretch for at least 30 seconds while doing it, if not slightly longer.

As you stretch, also remember to breathe deeply as this will help to loosen the muscles further and really allow you to move into that deep stretch as you should.

So there you have some of the top recovery strategies that you must be paying attention to as you go about your intense workouts.

You don't necessarily have to make use of every single one of them, but if you can make good use of at least two or three, you will notice a marked difference in how well this is influencing your ability to recover and feel well between sessions.

Different people will respond to some strategies better than others, so try out a few and see what works best for you.

So now that we've talked about what to do in order to prevent overtraining from occurring, what should you do if you're already in a state of overtraining?

What if you've pushed the barrier too far and now you're in dire need to get out of it?

In this case, action must be taken to reverse the situation and ensure that it doesn't happen again.

Let's go over your recovery protocol to get over overtraining.

What To Do If You're Overtrained

If you've found yourself in the position of being overtrained, you're likely feeling a little anxious and scared of what's to come next.

For many people in this situation, the instant fear is that they're going to have to stop training, which is not only going to cause them to lose all the fitness gains that they've worked so hard to achieve all this time, but that they're also going to be adding more body fat again as well.

As you can imagine, this is something that definitely isn't desirable given how intensely you have been training.

Fortunately, that doesn't necessarily have to be the outcome. If you're catching overtraining in its earlier stages, chances are that with proper care, you can remedy the situation and get back to your training relatively quickly, so a loss of fitness won't be a concern.

If you're deep into overtraining, it may take a bit more time to work through this, therefore you may notice that you suffer a slight decrease in your fitness level.

But, you have to weigh things overall. You could keep going as is, performing less than optimally and dig yourself deeper into the hole, or you could rest up, get better, and then be smarter with your training and get on the road to some real results.

Which would you prefer?

When you think rationally and without fear standing in your way, you see the second option is far better. So take care of yourself now so that you'll be in a better position, not a worse one, tomorrow.

Let's look at what you need to do.

Immediate Action

First things first, you need to take immediate action. If you have a number of the symptoms of overtraining and they have been occurring for a continuous 7-10 period (or longer), this isn't a time to play games.

Don't think that you'll cut back slightly and see how you feel in another week. At this point your body is crying for help and while cutting back is good, it's not fixing the situation. You're essentially just decreasing the extent of the further damage that is going to take place.

Nothing short of pure, 100% rest is going to help get you moving in the right direction again.

So your immediate course of action is to stop all workouts. Yes, it will be hard and you're likely going to fight some feelings of anxiety while doing so, but this is a must. There is no way around it.

Also, fight the urge to get out and go for a 'walk'. Many of those type A behavior people who are dead set on getting results will try and use this as an excuse just to get moving – just a little bit.

But, that easy going walk they set out on to get some fresh air soon turns into a powerwalk and before they know it, they're doing a workout session.

Rest – meaning relaxing on the couch and taking care of your body is what you're after.

The next thing that you need to be doing is looking after your nutrition as well. Here you have to assess where you were and what you need to do.

If you were dieting intensely before, this could be, in part, a reason why you are overtrained at this point. If this is the case, you're going to need to increase your calorie intake, especially your carbohydrates.

 Get an Edge!
If you are suffering from overtraining, it is very critical that you stop dieting immediately. Continuing to diet while you are overtrained is the biggest recipe for disaster as it will instantly make it next to impossible for you to recover.

Again, you'll fight some mental resistance with this. You immediately will think you're going to gain back a bunch of fat and will talk yourself out of following through with this. You must avoid this though.

One of the key things that you need to be doing right now to get yourself out of overtraining is restoring your muscle glycogen levels. Low muscle glycogen levels coupled with intense physical activity is a sure-fire recipe for overtraining, so your primary objective is fixing this.

You don't need to go crazy with your carbohydrate intake, but consuming around 150-200 grams per day would be a very wise move. Your dietary fat intake can be reduced slightly to help accommodate to the extra calories if you are very stressed out about the potential of weight gain.

Even still though, avoid bringing the calories too low. Your body needs energy right now to heal itself so if you adopt a super-low calorie intake, you're not going to be providing this energy at all. Moving to maintenance at this point, which is around 14-15 calories per pound of body weight would be a smart move.

Keep in mind you may gain some temporary weight from the extra water that comes on with the muscle glycogen storage you'll get, but this will be lost quickly once you're healed and start exercising again. Do not stress about this.

Now, the other scenario is where you weren't dieting at all but were just doing too much exercise. If that's the case, then as you move into this rest period to recover from overtraining, you'll want to cut back on your calorie intake slightly.

The reason being that if you were eating to meet your needs before, now that you aren't doing any of those intense workout sessions, your calorie needs will be lower.

Again, don't cut them back too much, but if you do want to prevent gaining body fat while you're resting, a 200-300 calorie reduction would be wise.

Still keep carbs high as they are required for good recovery, but decrease them in proportion to the other nutrients to achieve a proper calorie intake.

Finally, the last thing that you need to be doing immediately is looking at your stress levels and reducing any and all stress as much as possible. Right now any stress is going to hinder your ability to get better so the lower it is, the faster this process will go.

Also start practicing some of the same recovery strategies we mentioned above (foam rolling, hot baths, massage, etc) during this time as well. This will help relax the body and improve your muscle's recovery.

How long you're going to have to wait before you get back to your workouts will really depend on just how severe the overtraining process was.

Most people will be looking at around 1-2 weeks of full rest before they slowly ease themselves back into it.

If you've been overtraining for quite some time though and have really dug yourself into a whole, then you may need to rest up for a full month (or even longer) until you're feeling 100% again.

It can take a while. If you've been pushing for 12 months straight without paying attention to what your body was telling you, you're going to have to pay the price right now for it.

This is why preventing overtraining in the first place is so critically important.

Now let's shift gears a little and look at what you should be doing once you are becoming fully recovered and want to ease back into things.

Moving Forward Into The Future

The very first thing that you must keep in mind as you move into the future is that you need to do so slowly.

Don't ever, after taking time off due to overtraining, just dive back into your workouts right where you left off.

Do this and you'll find yourself quickly overtrained again and back right where you were.

First, you may have lost a little bit of fitness, so easing into things will help your body adapt again to the physical demands that the exercise is calling for.

Secondly, by easing back into things, you can better assess your tolerance for exercise and ensure that you are in fact recovered.

If you begin your workouts again and find that after just a couple you're facing the same symptoms you were when you first realized you needed time off, this indicates that you are not fully recovered yet and more time off is likely necessary.

You should be taking about 2-4 weeks of this gradual progression with your workouts to get back to the level you were at before.

Don't rush the process because doing so will hinder your results.

The second thing that you need to be doing as you move back to your workout program is taking a good hard look at that workout program itself. Try and figure out why it was that you become overtrained in the first place.

In some cases the reason will be clear – maybe you just had too much stress going on in your life and failed to look after your nutritional needs. In that case, the solution would be simple and moving forward, you'd just have to make sure to limit your stress and eat properly.

If it was something else however – training related, then you're going to have to make some program adjustments.

Maybe the workout sessions you were doing were just a little too much for your body and now that you're ready to get going again, you're going to have to cut back on them slightly.

Make sure that you are doing a full evaluation of every element of your program plan.

So this now brings us to a close on what you must be doing in order to prevent overtraining from occurring. Hopefully you now have a very good idea moving forwards how to approach your workout sessions so that you can see results and not be left feeling wiped, lacking progress, and frustrated with how things are progressing.

Do not overlook the criticalness of overtraining. If you do, you will find yourself in the position where you will have to deal with it.

This now brings us to a close on the second section of this book, so now let's move into part three, which is your section for action.

Part 3

CHAPTER 16:
Your Sample Meal Plans

Now it's time to show you your meal plan chart. What you're doing to do for this chart is find your calorie intake listed below and then follow the meal plan along with the servings of food listed.

Find the foods on the meal food chart below that to create your own unique meals that will help you stick to a healthy diet and feel as satisfied as possible.

You are free to choose any food listed under each category, but don't cross-mix categories (choose a carb rather than a protein for instance).

Meal/Calories	1600 1700 1800 1900	2000 2100 2200 2300	2400 2500 2600 2700	2800 2900 3000 3100	3200 3300 3400 3500
Breakfast	1 protein 1 carb 1 fruit 1 fat 1 vegetable	1 protein 1 carb 1 fruit 1 fat 1 vegetables	1 protein 1 carb 1 carb 1 fruit 1 fat 1 vegetables	1 protein 1 carb 1 carb 1 fruit 1 fat 1 vegetables	2 protein 2 carb 1 fruit 1 fat 1 vegetables
Mid-Morning	1 protein 1 fruit	1 protein 1 carb 1 fat	1 protein 1 carb 1 fat	1 protein 2 carb 1 fat	1 protein 2 carb 1 fruit 1 fat
Lunch	1 protein 1 carb 1 fat 2 vegetables	1 protein 2 carb 1 fat 1 vegetable	1 protein 1 protein 2 carb 1 fat 1 vegetable	1 protein 1 protein 2 carb 1 fat 1 vegetable	2 protein 2 carb 1 fat 1 fat 1 vegetable
Mid-Afternoon	1 protein 1 fat	1 protein 1 carb 1 fat	1 protein 1 carb 1 fat 1 fruit	1 protein 1 carb 1 fat 1 fruit	1 protein 1 carb 1 fat 1 fruit
Dinner	1 protein 1 fat 2 vegetables	1 protein 1 carb 1 carb 1 fat 2 vegetable	1 protein 1 carb 1 carb 1 fat 2 vegetable	1 protein 1 protein 1 carb 1 fat 2 vegetable	2 protein 1 carb 1 fat 2 vegetable
Before Bed	1 protein 1 fat	1 protein 1 fat	1 protein 1 fat	1 protein 1 fat 1 fat	1 protein 2 fat
Pre-Workout*	1 protein 1 carb	1 protein 1 carb	1 protein 1 carb	1 protein 1 carb	1 protein 1 carb 1 carb
Post-Workout**	1 protein 1 carb	1 protein 1 carb	1 protein 1 carb	1 protein 3 carb	1 protein 3 carb

Food Choices Chart

Protein Rich Food	One Serving Size**	Carb Rich Food	Serving Size	Fat Rich Food	Serving Size
Chicken breast	89 gms	Quinoa	½ cup cooked	Olive oil	1 tbsp
Turkey breast	89 gms	Brown rice	½ cup cooked	Sunflower oil	1 tbsp
White fish	118 gms	Barley	½ cup cooked	Safflower oil	1 tbsp
Eggs	2 eggs	Oatmeal	¼ cup (raw measurement)	Flaxseed oil	1 tbsp
Salmon	89 gms (also counts as 1 fat)	Whole wheat tortilla	1 small	Flaxseeds	2 tbsp
Lean red meat	89 gms	Whole wheat pita	1 small	Natural peanut butter	1 tbsp
Canned tuna	1 can	Whole grain bread	1 slice	Almond butter	1 tbsp
Whey protein powder	1 scoop	Bran/whole grain cereal	½-1 cup (check box for serving size)	Almonds	10
Tofu	89 gms	Whole wheat pasta	½ cup	Pecans	10
		Sweet potato	1 small	Sesame/ Poppyseeds	1 tbsp
		Whole grain crackers	5-10 depending on size	Avocado	½ cup sliced
				Salmon/fatty fish	3 oz (counts as 1 protein as well)
Dairy Rich Food	**One Serving Size****	**Fruits/Vegetables**	**One Serving Size****		
Cottage cheese	Cottage cheese	Fruit (apples, oranges, banana, pear)	1 piece		
Greek yogurt/low-fat yogurt	½ cup	Berries and melons	1 cup		
		Vegetables	1-2 cups*		

CHAPTER 17

Your 8 Week Beginner Workout Program

Week 1
Workout 1

Exercise	Reps	Sets	Rest
Squats	8	3	90 seconds
Bench Press	8	3	90 seconds
Deadlifts	8	3	90 seconds
Bent Over Rows	8	3	90 seconds
Shoulder Press	10	2	60 seconds
Bicep Curls	12	2	30 seconds
Tricep Extensions	12	2	30 seconds
Plank Hold	60 seconds	2	30 seconds

Workout 2

Exercise	Reps	Sets	Rest
Leg Press	8	3	90 seconds
Incline Bench Press	8	3	90 seconds
Step-ups	8	3	90 seconds
Pull-Ups	8	3	90 seconds
Single Arm Rows	10	2	60 seconds
Lateral Raises	12	2	30 seconds
Front Raises	12	2	30 seconds
Reverse Crunch	12	2	30 seconds

Workout 3

Exercise	Reps	Sets	Rest
Sumo Squats	8	3	90 seconds
Decline Bench Press	8	3	90 seconds
Lunges	8	3	90 seconds
Bent Over Rows	8	3	90 seconds
Shoulder Press	10	2	60 seconds
Hammer Bicep Curls	12	2	30 seconds
Dips	12	2	30 seconds
Lying Leg Raise	12	2	30 seconds

Week 2
Workout 1

Exercise	Reps	Sets	Rest
Squats	8	4	90 seconds
Bench Press	8	4	90 seconds
Deadlifts	8	4	90 seconds
Bent Over Rows	8	4	90 seconds
Shoulder Press	10	2	60 seconds
Bicep Curls	12	2	30 seconds
Tricep Extensions	12	2	30 seconds
Plank Hold	60 seconds	2	30 seconds

Workout 2

Exercise	Reps	Sets	Rest
Leg Press	8	4	90 seconds
Incline Bench Press	8	4	90 seconds
Step-ups	8	4	90 seconds
Pull-Ups	8	4	90 seconds
Single Arm Rows	10	2	60 seconds
Lateral Raises	12	2	30 seconds
Front Raises	12	2	30 seconds
Reverse Crunch	12	2	30 seconds

Workout 3

Exercise	Reps	Sets	Rest
Sumo Squats	8	4	90 seconds
Decline Bench Press	8	4	90 seconds
Lunges	8	4	90 seconds
Bent Over Rows	8	4	90 seconds
Shoulder Press	10	2	60 seconds
Hammer Bicep Curls	12	2	30 seconds
Dips	12	2	30 seconds
Lying Leg Raise	12	2	30 seconds

Week 3
Workout 1

Exercise	Reps	Sets	Rest
Squats	5	5	2 minutes
Bench Press	5	5	2 minutes
Deadlifts	5	5	2 minutes
Bent Over Rows	5	3	2 minutes
Shoulder Press	10	2	60 seconds
Bicep Curls	12	1	30 seconds
Tricep Extensions	12	1	30 seconds
Plank Hold	60 seconds	1	30 seconds

Workout 2

Exercise	Reps	Sets	Rest
Leg Press	5	5	2 minutes
Incline Bench Press	5	5	2 minutes
Step-ups	5	5	2 minutes
Pull-Ups	8	2	90 seconds
Single Arm Rows	10	2	60 seconds
Lateral Raises	12	1	30 seconds
Front Raises	12	1	30 seconds
Reverse Crunch	12	1	30 seconds

Workout 3

Exercise	Reps	Sets	Rest
Sumo Squats	5	5	90 seconds
Decline Bench Press	5	5	90 seconds
Lunges	8	4	90 seconds
Bent Over Rows	8	4	90 seconds
Shoulder Press	12	2	60 seconds
Hammer Bicep Curls	15	2	30 seconds
Dips	15	2	30 seconds
Lying Leg Raise	60 seconds	4	30 seconds

Week 4 (deloading week – reduced volume to allow for full recovery before moving forward for the second half of the workout program)

Workout 1

Exercise	Reps	Sets	Rest
Squats	5	2	2 minutes
Bench Press	5	2	2 minutes
Deadlifts	5	2	2 minutes
Bent Over Rows	5	2	2 minutes
Shoulder Press	10	1	60 seconds
Plank Hold	60 seconds	1	30 seconds

Workout 2

Exercise	Reps	Sets	Rest
Leg Press	5	2	2 minutes
Incline Bench Press	5	2	2 minutes
Step-ups	5	2	2 minutes
Pull-Ups	8	2	90 seconds
Single Arm Rows	10	1	60 seconds
Reverse Crunch	12	1	30 seconds

Workout 3

Exercise	Reps	Sets	Rest
Sumo Squats	5	2	90 seconds
Decline Bench Press	5	2	90 seconds
Lunges	8	2	90 seconds
Bent Over Rows	8	2	90 seconds
Shoulder Press	12	2	60 seconds
Lying Leg Raise	60 seconds	2	30 seconds

Week 5
Workout 1

Exercise	Reps	Sets	Rest
Squats	8	3	60 seconds
Bench Press	8	3	60 seconds
Deadlifts	8	3	60 seconds
Bent Over Rows	8	3	60 seconds
Shoulder Press	10	3	60 seconds
Bicep Curls	12	3	30 seconds
Tricep Extensions	12	3	30 seconds
Plank Hold	60 seconds	3	30 seconds

Workout 2

Exercise	Reps	Sets	Rest
Leg Press	8	3	60 seconds
Incline Bench Press	8	3	60 seconds
Step-ups	8	3	60 seconds
Pull-Ups	8	3	60 seconds
Single Arm Rows	10	3	60 seconds
Lateral Raises	12	3	30 seconds
Front Raises	12	3	30 seconds
Reverse Crunch	12	3	30 seconds

Workout 3

Exercise	Reps	Sets	Rest
Sumo Squats	8	3	60 seconds
Decline Bench Press	8	3	60 seconds
Lunges	8	3	60 seconds
Bent Over Rows	8	3	60 seconds
Shoulder Press	10	3	60 seconds
Hammer Bicep Curls	12	3	30 seconds
Dips	12	3	30 seconds
Lying Leg Raise	12	3	30 seconds

Week 6
Workout 1

Exercise	Reps	Sets	Rest
Squats	8	4	60 seconds
Bench Press	8	4	60 seconds
Deadlifts	8	4	60 seconds
Bent Over Rows	8	4	60 seconds
Shoulder Press	10	2	60 seconds
Bicep Curls	12	2	30 seconds
Tricep Extensions	12	2	30 seconds
Plank Hold	60 seconds	2	30 seconds

Workout 2

Exercise	Reps	Sets	Rest
Leg Press	8	4	60 seconds
Incline Bench Press	8	4	60 seconds
Step-ups	8	4	60 seconds
Pull-Ups	8	4	60 seconds
Single Arm Rows	10	2	60 seconds
Lateral Raises	12	2	30 seconds
Front Raises	12	2	30 seconds
Reverse Crunch	12	2	30 seconds

Workout 3

Exercise	Reps	Sets	Rest
Sumo Squats	8	4	60 seconds
Decline Bench Press	8	4	60 seconds
Lunges	8	4	60 seconds
Bent Over Rows	8	4	60 seconds
Shoulder Press	10	2	60 seconds
Hammer Bicep Curls	12	2	30 seconds
Dips	12	2	30 seconds
Lying Leg Raise	12	2	30 seconds

Week 7
Workout 1

Exercise	Reps	Sets	Rest
Squats	5	5	2 minutes
Bench Press	5	5	2 minutes
Deadlifts	5	5	2 minutes
Bent Over Rows	5	3	2 minutes
Shoulder Press	10	2	60 seconds
Bicep Curls	12	2	30 seconds
Tricep Extensions	12	2	30 seconds
Plank Hold	60 seconds	2	30 seconds

Workout 2

Exercise	Reps	Sets	Rest
Leg Press	5	5	2 minutes
Incline Bench Press	5	5	2 minutes
Step-ups	5	5	2 minutes
Pull-Ups	8	2	90 seconds
Single Arm Rows	10	2	60 seconds
Lateral Raises	12	2	30 seconds
Front Raises	12	2	30 seconds
Reverse Crunch	12	2	30 seconds

Workout 3

Exercise	Reps	Sets	Rest
Sumo Squats	5	5	90 seconds
Decline Bench Press	5	5	90 seconds
Lunges	8	4	90 seconds
Bent Over Rows	8	4	90 seconds
Shoulder Press	12	2	60 seconds
Hammer Bicep Curls	15	2	30 seconds
Dips	15	2	30 seconds
Lying Leg Raise	60 seconds	4	30 seconds

Week 8 (deloading week – reduced volume to allow for full recovery before moving forward for the intermediate program)

Workout 1

Exercise	Reps	Sets	Rest
Squats	5	2	2 minutes
Bench Press	5	2	2 minutes
Deadlifts	5	2	2 minutes
Bent Over Rows	5	2	2 minutes
Shoulder Press	10	1	60 seconds
Plank Hold	60 seconds	1	30 seconds

Workout 2

Exercise	Reps	Sets	Rest
Leg Press	5	2	2 minutes
Incline Bench Press	5	2	2 minutes
Step-ups	5	2	2 minutes
Pull-Ups	8	2	90 seconds
Single Arm Rows	10	1	60 seconds
Reverse Crunch	12	1	30 seconds

Workout 3

Exercise	Reps	Sets	Rest
Sumo Squats	5	2	90 seconds
Decline Bench Press	5	2	90 seconds
Lunges	8	2	90 seconds
Bent Over Rows	8	2	90 seconds
Shoulder Press	12	2	60 seconds
Lying Leg Raise	60 seconds	2	30 seconds

CHAPTER 18:
Your 8 Week Intermediate/Advanced Workout Program

The following is the 8 week advanced workout program and is designed to utilize the advanced concepts that we talked about earlier. As you move through this protocol you may notice higher than normal levels of fatigue, so be sure that you are practicing the proper recovery strategies that we talked about during the overtraining section.

Week 1 – Superset Week
Day 1:

Exercise	Sets	Reps	Rest
Superset: Squats And Bench Press	3	10-12	45 seconds
Superset: Deadlift And Bent Over Row	3	10-12	45 seconds
Shoulder Press	3	10	45 seconds
Lat Pull-Down	2	10	45 seconds
Standing Calf Raise	2	12	30 seconds

Day 2:

Exercise	Sets	Reps	Rest
Squats	3	8	60 seconds
Bench Press	3	8	60 seconds
Superset: Lunge And Shoulder Press	3	10	60 seconds
Superset: Bicep Curl And Tricep Extension	2	12	30 seconds
Lateral Raises	2	12	30 seconds
Plank	3	45-60 second hold	30 seconds

Day 3:

Exercise	Sets	Reps	Rest
Superset: Step-Ups And Push-Ups	3	20	60 seconds
Superset: Deadlift And Pull-Ups	3	15/20	60 seconds
Shoulder Press	3	10	60 seconds
Lunges	3	10	60 seconds
Standing Calf Raises	2	15	30 seconds

Week 2 – Triset Week

Day 1:

Exercise	Sets	Reps	Rest
Triset: Squats, Bench Press, Tricep Extension	3	8	90 seconds
Triset: Deadlift, Bent Over Row, Bicep Curl	3	8	90 seconds
Shoulder Press	4	10	60 seconds
Plank Exercise	2	30-60 second hold	30 seconds

Day 2:

Exercise	Sets	Reps	Rest
Triset: Lunges, Push-Ups, Tricep Dips	3	15	90 seconds
Triset: Step-Ups, Pull-Ups, Bicep Curls	3	10-15	90 seconds
Shoulder Press	4	10	60 seconds
Hamstring Curl	3	10	30 seconds
Standing Calf Raise	3	15	30 seconds

Day 3:

Exercise	Sets	Reps	Rest
Squats	8	4	60 seconds
Bench Press	8	4	60 seconds
Bent Over Rows	8	4	60 seconds
Shoulder Press	10	4	60 seconds
Triset: Bicep Curls, Tricep Extensions, Lateral Raise	12	2	60 seconds
Triset: Lying Leg Raise, Supermans, Reverse Crunch	12	2	60 seconds

Week 3 – Drop Set Week
<u>Day 1:</u>

Exercise	Sets	Reps	Rest
Bench Press	3	8	60 seconds
Squats	3	8	60 seconds
Deadlifts	3	8	60 seconds
Bent over Rows	3	8	60 seconds
Drop Set: Shoulder Press	1	10-10-10	45 seconds
Drop set: Bicep Curls	1	12-12-12	45 seconds
Plank	2	60 seconds	30 seconds

<u>Day 2:</u>

Exercise	Sets	Reps	Rest
Incline Bench Press	3	12	45 seconds
Lunges	3	12	45 seconds
Shoulder Press	3	12	45 seconds
Step-Ups	3	12	45 seconds
Drop Set: Bent Over Rows	1	10-10-10	45 seconds
Drop set: Tricep Extension	1	12-12-12	45 seconds
Lying Leg Raise	2	15	30 seconds

<u>Day 3:</u>

Exercise	Sets	Reps	Rest
Squats	4	8	60 seconds
Bent Over Rows	4	8	60 seconds
Deadlifts	4	8	60 seconds
Drop Set: Bench Press	1	8-8-8	60 seconds
Drop Set: Standing Calf Raise	1	12-12-12	30 seconds
Lateral Raise	2	10	45 seconds

Week 4: Pyramid Sets
Day 1:

Exercise	Sets	Reps	Rest
Bench Press	5	6-8-10-8-6	60 seconds
Squats	5	6-8-10-8-6	60 seconds
Bent Over Rows	5	6-8-10-8-6	60 seconds
Plank Exercise	3	60 second hold	60 seconds
Shoulder Press	3	10	60 seconds
Lunges	3	12	60 seconds

Day 2:

Exercise	Sets	Reps	Rest
Incline Bench Press	5	8-10-12-10-8	60 seconds
Deadlifts	5	6-8-10-8-6	60 seconds
Pull-Downs	5	8-10-12-10-8	60 seconds
Calf Raises	3	15	60 seconds
Bicep Curls	3	12	45 seconds
Tricep Extensions	3	12	45 seconds

Day 3:

Exercise	Sets	Reps	Rest
Bench Press	5	6-8-10-8-6	60 seconds
Squats	5	6-8-10-8-6	60 seconds
Bent Over Row	5	6-8-10-8-6	60 seconds
Lateral Raise	3	12	45 seconds
Lying leg Raise	3	12	45 seconds

*You'll notice that these workouts are slightly shorter in terms of total exercises performed and this is to account for the higher sets performed on the pyramid sets.

Do not add additional exercises to these sessions because you don't feel as though there is enough included. This will only lead to you becoming quickly overtrained.

Week 5: Pre-Fatigue Set Workout

Day 1:

Exercise	Sets	Reps	Rest
Tricep Extension	2	12	30 seconds
Bench Press	4	8	60 seconds
Leg Extension	2	12	30 seconds
Lunges	4	8	60 seconds
Bent Over Row	4	8	60 seconds
Hamstring Curl	2	12	30 seconds

Day 2:

Exercise	Sets	Reps	Rest
Bicep Curl	2	12	30 seconds
Bent Over Row	4	8	60 seconds
Hamstring Curl	2	12	30 seconds
Deadlift	4	8	60 seconds
Leg Extension	2	12	30 seconds
Shoulder Press	3	12	60 seconds

Day 3:

Exercise	Sets	Reps	Rest
Lateral Raise	2	12	30 seconds
Shoulder Press	4	8	60 seconds
Hamstring Curl	2	12	30 seconds
Squats	4	8	60 seconds
Bench Press	4	8	60 seconds
Bent Over Row	4	8	60 seconds

Week Six: Circuit Training Week
Day 1:
Perform the following exercises all in a row, taking no break between them. Aim to complete 8-10 reps each. Once they're all finished, rest for 60 seconds and then repeat three more times through.

Squats
Reverse Crunch
Bench Press
Split Squats
Lying Leg Raise
Bent Over Row
Shoulder Press
Plank

Day 2:
Perform the following exercises all in a row, taking no break between them. Aim to perform as many reps as you can in a one minute time frame. Once they're all finished, rest for 60 seconds and then repeat one more time through.

Squats
Crunch On The Ball
Push-Ups On The Ball
Burpees
Shoulder Press On The Ball
Supermans
Single Leg Deadlifts
Pull-Ups
Side Plank
Jumping Jacks

Day 3:

Perform the following exercises all in a row, taking no break between them. Aim to complete 20 reps each. Once they're all finished, rest for 60 seconds and then repeat one more time through.

Step-Ups
Pull-Ups
Bicycle
Jump Lunges
Bench Press
Mountain Climbers
Calf Raises
Shoulder Press
Bicep Curls
Tricep Extension

Week Seven: Timed Set Week

Perform the following circuit training workouts, doing each exercise for one minute and aiming to perform as many reps as possible in each minute. Once each circuit is finished, repeat one more time through.

Day 1
Push-Ups
Squats
Bent Over Rows
Lunges
Reverse Crunch
Shoulder Press
Burpees

Day 2
Chest Press
Step-Ups
Bicep Curls
Lying Leg Raise
Overhead Tricep Extension
Deadlifts

Day 3
Incline Chest Press
Squats
Pull-Downs
Lunges
Reverse Crunch
Lateral Raise
Front Raise
Plank Hold

Week Eight: Back Off Week (to allow for rest and recovery before repeating the cycle once again).

<u>Day 1:</u>

Exercise	Sets	Reps	Rest
Chest Press	2	8	2 minutes
Squats	2	8	2 minutes
Bent Over Rows	2	8	2 minutes
Deadlifts	2	8	2 minutes
Shoulder Press	2	8	1 minute
Plank	2	60 seconds	1 minute

<u>Day 2:</u>

Exercise	Sets	Reps	Rest
Incline Chest Press	2	8	2 minutes
Step ups	2	8	2 minutes
Bent Over Rows	2	8	2 minutes
Leg Press	2	8	2 minutes
Lat Pull-Down	2	8	1 minute
Reverse Crunch	2	15	1 minute

<u>Day 3:</u>

Exercise	Sets	Reps	Rest
Chest Press	2	8	2 minutes
Squats	2	8	2 minutes
Bent Over Rows	2	8	2 minutes
Deadlifts	2	8	2 minutes
Shoulder Press	2	8	1 minute
Lying Leg Raise	2	10	1 minute

CHAPTER 19:
Your Pressed-For-Time Workout Solution

Finally, to finish things off we have your pressed-for-time workout solution. The following workouts are going to be just ten minutes in length so will be ideal for those of you who for whatever reason are unable to get your full workout in.

Simply do these and you will maintain your level of fitness while you are unable to get to the gym as often as you would have liked.

Make note that these workouts are not going to be ideal for seeing ongoing and constant progression, however they can be a great way to keep yourself from losing fitness during an especially busy period of your life or a time when you just aren't as motivated.

If you can get yourself to do these workouts, which will take around 10-15 minutes, you can still keep your strength up, which will then easily allow you to move forward when you are ready.

Make sure that you give 100% to these workout sessions as it's your ongoing effort that will ensure they are going to be as effective as they need to be despite only being such a short session.

Workout A
Perform 10 reps of the following exercises, taking about 30 seconds of rest between each exercise. Lift a heavy enough weight that you are fully fatigued by the time that you're finished the last and final rep.

Squats
Bench Press
Deadlifts
Bent Over Row
Shoulder Press
Bicep Curl
Tricep Extension
Reverse Crunch
Plank Exercise

Workout B
Perform 3 sets of 5 reps of each of the following exercises, taking 1 minute rest between each set.

Squats
Bench Press
Bent Over Rows
Lunges

Workout C

Perform the following circuit, taking no rest in between each exercise and doing as many reps as you can for one minute.

Burpees
Push-Ups
Walking Lunges
Chair Dips
Plank Hold (1 minute)
Mountain Climbers
Bodyweight Sumo Squats
Shoulder Press
Pull-Ups
Jumping Jacks

Workout D

Perform the following supersets, doing 12 reps of each exercise and taking 30 seconds rest between each superset. Do one superset total before moving on to the next.

Squats with Bench Press
Deadlift with Bent Over Row
Lunge with Shoulder Press
Bicep Curl with Tricep Extension
Lateral Raise With Front Raise

Alternate between the workouts or choose whichever strikes your fancy as you need in order to stay the course on the plan. Just keep in mind that even though these workouts are short, you will still need to take one day off between them as they are still utilizing that full body approach that will require the day between for rest and recovery purposes.

Conclusion

So there you have your complete guide to getting into the best shape of your life, improving your health, and continuing on to lead a healthier and more fulfilling lifestyle in the long run.

Make sure that you take things at your own pace as you move along with this program. Remember that change doesn't happen overnight and for some people, it will take longer to stay committed and make the changes they need to than others.

Be patient with yourself as you go about this process. If you're patient and let things progress as they should, you will see great long term results. If you press it and try and force yourself to do things you aren't quite comfortable and ready for yet or you're just going to get frustrated and fall off the bandwagon.

Instead be smart, progress at a pace that's right for you doing things that you enjoy. If you do this, you will be creating a new lifestyle that you can comfortably stick with over time.

About the author

Shannon Clark holds a degree in Exercise Science from the University of Alberta, where she specialized in Sports Performance and Psychology. In addition to her degree, she is an AFLCA certified personal trainer and has been working in the field for over 8 years now.

She is a regular contributor to Bodybuilding.com and has also been named 'Writer Of The Year' two times running. She has been featured in the Iron Man magazine and has contributed well over 400 articles to a variety of different websites dedicated towards muscle building and athletic performance.

Shannon has spent the better part of her adult years researching and studying the top methods to build lean muscle as well as achieve maximum states of leanness. She currently works with a variety of different clients with various goal sets, helping them reach whatever physique goals they have set for themselves.

Finally, amongst all her research she's also made a test subject of herself trying out many of the different training and diet techniques she's come across. From Ketogenic diets to Intermittent Fasting protocols, she's always anxious to find out what type of results the latest protocols will deliver.

In her spare time, she enjoys reading, experimenting with new recipes, weight lifting, and hiking.

www.ingramcontent.com/pod-product-compliance
Lightning Source LLC
Chambersburg PA
CBHW082130290526
45794CB00008B/2984